FREESTYLE
INSTANT
POT
Cookbook

First Published in 2018 by Sally Walker

ISBN-13: 978-1720765547
ISBN-10: 1720765545

Interior, Front and Back Cover Design by Sally Walker.

Printed in the United States of America.

First Edition

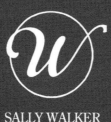

SALLY WALKER

CONTENTS

Beef Recipes

Chicken Recipes

Pork Recipes

Sides Dishes and Snacks Recipes

7

Dessert Recipes

AUTHOR

"To my dearest Simon"

A graduate of New York University, Sally Walker earned her bachelor's degree in Health and Nutrition in 1989. She then worked as a professional—much loved—dietitian in hospitals throughout California and the East Coast. After a highly successful career helping millions of people lose weight, Sally has now gracefully retired to Los Angeles, CA. Every month Sally likes to give something back to society by hosting Weight Watchers diet classes to help people lose weight in her local community. In her precious free time, Sally likes cooking, blogging, walking and spending time with friends and family.

.... Sally

Freestyle 101

Freestyle 101

<u>What is Weight Watchers?</u>

Weight Watchers! You may have heard these two words spoken now and then, whether it's in everyday conversation, on the TV or online. Weight Watchers is a buzzword for 'diet' or 'dieting'. It is an excellent diet for people wanting to lose weight and achieve a healthy and more proactive lifestyle. While you can certainly lose up to two pounds every week, Weight Watchers believe that there is more to losing weight than simply counting calories—it has evolved to include flexibility and choice to suit your everyday dieting needs. The team behind the Weight Watchers diet believe that everyone can choose to substitute unhealthy foods with healthy foods—and by doing so, change your behavior and your body too. Today, there is a wide variety of Weight Watchers programs designed to help people eat better, exercise more, and transform themselves into the person they want to be—to live a healthy and long life.

One of the most iconic and important part of Weight Watchers is its point system. When Weight Watchers first started, for example, they used a point system based on an exchange diet, which was a lot more restrictive than the new SmartPoints system released in early 2018. Today, all foods are assigned SmartPoints based on the nutritional content of the food. In works like this: foods high in sugar and saturated fat are assigned higher SmartPoints values, while foods high in protein will decrease the SmartPoints value. So, foods that keep you fuller for longer "cost" the least SmartPoints, while foods that are nutritionally dense will cost less than foods with minimal calories. This means that if you are given the option of a chicken salad sandwich or lobster bisque soup, both have 380 calories, but the sandwich would be a smarter choice.

The great thing about the Weight Watchers is that their diets are structured to perfection, allowing you the most amount of freedom, support and success. The SmartPoints system is based on a multi-model approach that allows people to access support groups, so they can share their experience and seek advice from others— this was what Weight Watchers founder Jean Nidetch did when she founded Weight Watchers. Today, the world has become more connected and digital, meaning you can access support via online chat, phone and chat forums— help is at the tip of your fingertips with only one click of your mouse! So, you now have the choice to follow the plan online if this is more suitable for you. But, it is worth keeping in mind that Weight Watchers did their own research and found that those who went to meetings and used their mobile app lost almost eight times more weight than those who go it alone.

Weight Watchers History

Weight Watchers was founded by homemaker, Jean Nidetch, at her house in Queens, New York, in 1963. It was here where Jean invited her friends round for coffee and chatted about her addiction to cookies! Today, Weight Watchers operates in 30 countries worldwide—but it took over 50 years to get here!

After Jean's meetings at Queens, she then went on to publish a book during the early 70s entitled *The Memoir of a Successful Loser the Story of Weight Watchers*. This book covered how the original plan for Weight Watchers worked and was later replaced with the *Weight Watchers Program Handbook for Ladies.* This new plan worked very much like the original.

In 1989, the plan then changed again to what was known as an exchange-based diet, which involved participants knowing the amount of food that they could eat from each food group. These groups included fats, fruit, dairy, and vegetables. For example, a "fat exchange" could be a tablespoon of olive oil. If your plan allowed you to exchange fats each day, then you could use two tablespoons of oil to dress your salad. This would exhaust your fat exchange for the entire day. Ultimately, this type of exchange was a different way to control calories.

In 1997, the first points program was introduced, called the 1-2-3 Success Program. This new system gave members an easy way to track their fat, fiber, and calorie consumption. This new points system became the most popular, and points have remained a big part of Weight Watchers since. They switched the plan up a bit again in the early 2000s and changed the name to Winning Points. A small modification to their plan over the years was to allow the member to earn points through exercise. This gave members a little incentive to get moving.

The *Turn Around Program* was then implemented. This change gave members the chance to pick between two very different plans. The *Core Program* consisted of picking healthy foods from a certain list. Their other option was the Flex Plan. This gave members the chance to eat whatever they wanted to if they kept track of their points and stayed within their limit. The Core Program was gotten rid of in 2009 when the Weight Watchers Momentum Plan was introduced. This plan worked to help members better understand how eating certain foods helped them to stop overeating.

The New Freestyle Plan

The Freestyle plan is Weight Watchers' revolution. After over 50 years of previous plans, the Freestyle plan takes all the good bits from these plans and puts them into one simple plan that uses the new SmartPoints system. It is important to note that all point values for foods have stayed the same, and no food item has gone up in points. In fact, some foods have gone down to zero points!

What is different about the Freestyle plan, however, is that members can roll over some of their points. This change was implemented because Weight Watchers recognized that people's eating habits on Monday tended to be much different than Saturdays, for example. So, rollovers give members the flexibility to use fewer points one day, which means that they can have up to four extras to roll over into their weekly bank for days when they need more points.

Probably the most important change the Freestyle plan has introduced is that it now has over 200 "zero-point" foods that don't have to be tracked—you can eat these as much as you like (within moderation, of course)! These foods include things like fish, eggs, skinless chicken breast and beans. After 50 years, Weight Watchers still prides itself on the fact that you can eat whatever you want—nothing is strictly forbidden!

You might be wondering how much effort you need to put into the Freestyle plan. Having spoken to thousands of members, the plan starts with medium difficulty, but drops to basic after a few weeks. It's designed to help you make easy changes to your eating habits, and it's flexible enough that anybody should can fit it into their life. Through this program, you are taught how to make tweaks to your lifestyle by learning how to create affordable and delicious healthy eating habits.

Ultimately, speaking from personal experience, the level of effort required on the Freestyle plan really depends on the person. You can make it as easy or as hard as you want to. For example, you learn how to shop for and cook healthy foods, and ways to dine out to help support your weight loss—these things can make it easier for you. Also, you won't ever have to buy packaged meals. The plan still uses FitPoints, which means that you can get credit for all your physical activity too.

The great thing is, no matter your dietary restrictions, you can follow the Weight Watchers Freestyle program. If you're vegan, vegetarian, limited fat or salt, dairy-free, and so on, you can follow this program—if you do have any form of medical ailment, however, I would advise you to speak to your GP before starting it. The last thing I would want you to do is start the diet, then start having any form of medical problem—it's better to be safe than sorry in my opinion.

Weight Watchers Meetings

"The meetings are a vital lifeline for any Weight Watchers dieter"— Sandy Monroe, Jacksonville, FL.

Sandy Monroe, a 35-year-old mother of two, started attending small group meetings at her local community center when she started the Weight Watchers diet back in 2012. At first, Sandy was little afraid of going because she thought she was too self-conscious to sit with other women who she thought were more attractive and more successful than her. Sandy couldn't have been more wrong! Sandy turned out to be the most successful woman at the meeting. And her reason for success? Competition! Sandy was determined not to let the city girls knock her confidence, with their successful high-flying jobs and mortgages to boot. So, she decided to outperform them. Week after week, she was the woman who had lost the most—sometimes as much as 10lbs! Her success is a shining example of how meetings instill in people the confidence and fighting spirit to get things done—to lose weight through a competitive, friendly, atmosphere.

Today, these meetings are still vitally important for dieting and weight loss success. They last on average 30 minutes— which is a nice and convenient amount of time for a busy mom's schedule. The meetings are led by a Weight Watchers leader—or coach— who went through the Weight Watches program earlier on in their lives and has worked hard to keep the weight off too. The great thing about the coach is that you can talk to them about anything—they are an open book. So, if you are unsure about anything or have teething problems after starting your diet plan, your coach will put these problems right for you. Think of them as your friend, not a figure of authority, and you will get the most help from them. As the saying goes, every question is a good question, and this is certainly the mindset you should have when starting any Weight Watchers diet plan.

Weight Watchers meetings also help you solve problems as part of a group too. Everyone has the chance to talk in meetings because Weight Watchers prides itself on promoting an equal and inclusive environment for all, one which brings people together from all walks of life united by one common goal: losing weight! In these meetings, you will discuss the most important part of your diet: your Weight Watchers diet plan. What's great about diet plans is that they help dieters eat foods lower in calories, sugar and saturated fats, but higher in the good stuff: protein. Sharing ideas with your fellow dieters can be an inspiring and thought-provoking experience. However, I completely understand that for some people this can be a challenging thing to do. If it is for you, I would advise you to speak to speak to a friend or family member to at least share your progress—a problem shared is a problem halved!

Weight Watchers offers a wide range of personalized membership packages best suited for your diet—which can be personalized online using the Weight Watchers app. As they come with no fixed period, you can choose to cancel them anytime. However, 99% of people who purchase one of these packages do not cancel it— they work! While these plans do cost money, the cost varies with different promotions, depending on if you want to attend meetings each week, have a coach, use only the online tools, and so on. What is certain, however, is that each new member will pay a starter fee of $20 (but sometimes changes with promotions). Then, they will pick the offer that works best for them. There are three main costs associated with each plan:

- ✓ Their OnlinePlus system starts at $3.99 per week

- ✓ Meetings plus the OnlinePlus system starts at $7.99 per week

- ✓ Personal coaching starts at $12.69 per week

It is worth saying that if you pay for multi-months up front, you will get a discount in monthly fees. All of this adds up to an amazing program that will help you to lose weight. Weight Watchers participants tend to lose more weight than those on Atkins, Slim Fat, and Eat Yourself Slim.

SmartPoints

The Freestyle plan uses a revolutionary counting system called SmartPoints. This is a science-based points system that assigns each food a certain number of points based on four things: protein, sugar, saturated fat and calories. The higher the number of SmartPoints a food has, the higher the amount of fat and sugar it contains. The reasoning behind this system is that studies have found eating less saturated fat and sugar, as well as more protein, is a proven way to lose weight.

The Smart Points system is an improvement of the traditional ProPoint counting method that makes it easier for you to keep track of the foods you can and cannot eat on the Freestyle plan. Essentially, it allows you to set a daily meal budget to plan what foods you will eat throughout the day, week and months ahead. Therefore, the SmartPoints system is all about *control* and *freedom* and gives you the widest and healthiest selection of foods available on your Freestyle diet.

When you sign up for the Weight Watchers program, you will be assigned a SmartPoints budget. SmartPoints make you think wisely about the foods you eat. For example, foods high in sugar and unhealthy fats are assigned more points than foods high in protein like fruits and vegetables.

Whether a food is assigned 0, 1, 2 or 3 points and so on depends on how many calories, saturated fat, sugar and protein is in it. Therefore, when assessing which food is right for your diet, you should check the nutritional content of food, making note of the number of calories, proteins, saturated fats, sugars in it – food labels found on the side or back of food packaging are a great way to find out this information. Protein decreases smart point values, while the other three increase values.

How do SmartPoints work?

It's straightforward! When you decide to join the Freestyle program, you will be asked information like your weight, height, gender and age. This information is used to calculate a customised SmartPoints budget that is just right for you—so don't worry if your friend's budget is different to yours! As you continue through the program, this number could go down. You don't need to worry though; it's formulated to make sure that you receive the right amount of nutrients.

The great thing about the SmartPoints method is that you are given two budgets: daily and weekly. The daily budget is stricter than the weekly budget because it is what you need to stick to for the Freestyle plan to be most effective in helping you lose weight. The weekly budget allows you to be more flexible because it allows occasional splurges and treats—in moderation— and is intended to be a safety net. You spend them a little each day, or you could save them for the weekend if you have something special going on. You could also choose not to use them at all—whatever works best for you. Important: your weekly allowance of SmartPoints doesn't roll over to the next week, so if you don't use them, you lose them—they reset every week!

SmartPoints and Me

As you lose weight, your SmartPoints number adjusts so you can continue to drop pounds. The point number that helps you lose weight initially may be too great when your body shrinks in size. A smaller body uses less energy, so it requires fewer points to continue to lose weight. When you reach your goal weight and switch to maintenance, your Weight Watchers SmartPoint target shifts slightly upwards to keep you from losing too much weight. This higher point value helps even out your energy balance, so you consume and expend relatively equal amounts to maintain your weight. Sustaining a successful weight loss requires you continue to make good food choices most of the time, though.

The best way to keep track of your SmartPoints is through the Weight Watchers app. It makes it easy to look up the points so that you know what you're eating. SmartPoints are not the same as calories. Calories only tell part of the story of how food impacts the body. If you eat 100 calories of cookies, you won't receive the same nutrients as you would from 100 calories of turkey, vegetables or tofu.

For example, each of these breakfasts all have 300 calories:

✓ Chocolate chip pancake with maple syrup.

✓ Egg, avocado, and ham on a light English muffin with a banana.

✓ Peanut and Greek yogurt parfait with berries.

But when looking at them on the SmartPoints system, they are very, very different. Their SmartPoints are:

✓ 11 SmartPoints.

✓ 6 SmartPoints.

✓ 3 SmartPoints, respectively.

The bottom line of SmartPoints is that counting calories without paying attention to nutrients isn't going to lead to a healthier eating pattern. SmartPoints takes everything into consideration!

PROS AND CONS OF FREESTYLE

As with anything in life, there are good and not so good parts. Weight Watchers understands that its Freestyle program isn't suited to everyone, whether that's because of health issues or personal choice. So, if you're still trying to decide if you want to join Weight Watchers Freestyle, here are some pros and cons to help you make that choice.

Pros

✓ There are no forbidden foods on the Freestyle plan—that's right. As discussed, the plan removes the restrictions on foods all the previous Weight Watchers plans had—moderation is key.

✓ Freestyle provides you with lifestyle education, cooking advice, nutritional tips and so many more benefits.

✓ Weight Watchers meetings foster inclusivity and allow you to bring children as young as 13, but you may have to ask your physician for approval first.

✓ You will achieve weight loss at a rate decided by you. If you consume foods with fewer SmartPoints, expect to achieve faster weight loss. However, weight loss varies from person to person because it depends on how fast your metabolism is and how your body adapts to the Freestyle program.

✓ Freestyle helps you learn portion control. One of the biggest causes of weight gain is oversized meal portions. With the Freestyle plan, you will eat the right amount of food for your body.

✓ Freestyle plan promotes exercise. When you are on your way to the Weight Watchers meetings, you are keeping active and losing weight in the process. The meetings encourage a proactive lifestyle too.

✓ Freestyle encourages home cooking. Gone are the days when you would return from work and order that takeaway or microwave foods. On the Freestyle plan, you will learn how to cook wholesome and healthy foods appropriate for your body.

✓ The Weight Watchers app syncs with some of the most popular fitness trackers, so you can monitor your weight loss progress on the go.

Cons

Even though Weight Watchers has worked well for many people, it may not work for everybody.

✓ Depending on your household income, the cost of the Freestyle plan might be expensive for you. If it is, you should put things into perspective. Think of it as a good investment because you will benefit from it for the rest of your life when you lose weight and your lifestyle changes for the better.

✓ Some people don't like the weekly group meetings. If you are shy and don't like sharing your experiences with other people, that is fine—there is no harm it that at all. However, I would refer you to Sandy Monroe's story at the beginning of this book for inspiration.

✓ You must participate in weekly weigh-ins. Now, some people like them, others hate them. If you have lost lots of weight, you might like to show off in front of your group members. This is good because it encourages competition and motivates others to try harder. However, if you really don't want to do it, you don't have to— they are not mandatory.

✓ Some people might get discouraged with their weekly progress. Again, perspective is key. Compare yourself to where you were when you started the Freestyle plan and where you want to be when you finish it. Record your weight loss down on a piece of paper—or on your phone app—for motivation and the 'you can do it' attitude!

✓ Counting SmartPoints might become become tedious for you. If you are not used to counting calories, counting SmartPoints might seem a little difficult. You should make note of your daily SmartPoints budget and eventually it will become second nature to you. If you are used to counting calories, then counting SmartPoints will be an easy transition for you.

All diets, including the Freestyle plan, have their bonuses and drawbacks. It's important to weigh everything up to figure out if this is the right choice for you.

FOODS TO EAT AND FOODS TO AVOID

With the Freestyle program, and pretty much every Weight Watchers program, you don't have to restrict yourself to what you can and can't eat: this revolutionary change has been discussed earlier on in this book. Still, some foods are better than others. You should try to include these foods in your plan wherever possible.

Foods to Eat

This list is by no means exhaustive. You can literally eat whatever you want on the Freestyle plan, but most of these foods have zero points. For a detailed list, visit the website.

- ✓ Nonfat unsweetened yogurt
- ✓ Vegetables
- ✓ Fruits
- ✓ Peas
- ✓ Corn
- ✓ Lentils
- ✓ Tofu
- ✓ Beans
- ✓ Eggs
- ✓ Shellfish
- ✓ Fish
- ✓ Skinless chicken breast
- ✓ Lean pork
- ✓ Lean beef
- ✓ Whole grain foods
- ✓ Coconut
- ✓ Avocado

Foods to Avoid

Even though you can eat what you want if you stay within your SmartPoints range, this is not quite true. There are some things you should avoid—but these things should be obvious to any dieter on any diet. These foods include:

- Flavored and sweetened yogurt – a seemingly healthy food can end up having as much sugar as a handful of M&Ms, especially if you go for the yogurt with Oreos or other candies in them.

- Syrup – A tasty sweet treat on your morning pancakes may be delicious, but it's packed full of sugar. Try going for real maple syrup or honey. They contain actual nutrients.

- Coffee creamer – Coffee is fine if you don't fill up most of your cup with cream and sugar. Try to switch to black coffee instead—and no sugar tea too.

- High-sugar breakfast cereals – Not all cereals are made the same. Some can be a healthy breakfast option, while others are loaded with sugar. Usually, the children's cereal is the unhealthiest, while adult cereal is aimed specifically at the dieting market.

- Soda – Who doesn't love the fizzy drink? The problem is all the sugar and empty calories that sodas contain. These refined carbs can ruin your weight loss. Diet sodas are pretty much just as bad as well. Even sugar free drinks contain aspartame and sweeteners, which have been scientifically proven to be as unhealthy as full sugar drinks. Drink sparingly. Pure water is your best friend here,

There are plenty more things you should try to avoid while trying to lose weight, but if you listen to your coach and your body, you will learn to make the best decisions for your body.

MAKING SENSE OF FATS

Since fats make up a large and important portion of the Freestyle plan, they are vital for staying healthy and in shape. But it is not just consuming fat this is crucial, but choosing the right fats is important as well! There can be a lot of confusion as to what fats are good, bad, and those which should be avoided when cooking with your Instant Pot. Here we will break down those good and bad fats.

GOOD FATS: The "good guy" fats that are a go in your diet are split up into four different categories:

1. Saturated Fats
2. Monounsaturated fats (MUFAs)
3. Polyunsaturated fats (PUFAs)
4. Trans fats (naturally occurring)

When it boils down to "what types of aspects are in what fats," you must remember that all fats in the world are created by a mixture of all the above types of fat but are categorized by which one is the most dominant. Here, we will break down each type of fat when it comes to consuming foods with your Instant Pot. This will help you to easily see them when you are making decisions about what to fuel your body and mind with.

SATURATED FATS: Saturated fats had a bad reputation for many years. They were viewed as terrible for the health of your heart, and we were taught to either avoid them or to decrease our consumption of them.

However, since then there have been various studies to prove this wrong and have shown no significant link between saturated fats, to the risk of heart disease. We have been consuming saturated fats for *thousands* of years. Considering this new information, there is a plethora of great benefits that come along with the inclusion of healthy saturated fats in your daily diet.

Several saturated fats include something we call "medium-chain triglycerides (MCTs)," which are found in items like coconut oil and small amounts of butter and palm oil. MCT can be digested simply and easily in the body. When we eat these MCT's, they pass through the liver and are utilized automatically as an energy source! This means they are superb in your diet if you want to lose weight or boost your physical performance.

Health benefits of saturated fats:
- ✓ Increase in the function of the immune system
- ✓ Better cholesterol levels, both HDL and LDL
- ✓ Better HDL to LDL cholesterol ratio
- ✓ Improved maintenance of bone density
- ✓ Rise of HDL (good) cholesterol to prevent LDL.
- ✓ Promotes the creation of cortisol and testosterone.

Best sources of saturated fats:
- ✓ Cocoa butter
- ✓ Coconut oil
- ✓ Cream
- ✓ Eggs
- ✓ Lard

MONOUNSATURATED FATS: Unlike saturated fats, monounsaturated fatty acids (MUFAs) have been a graciously accepted "good fat" for a long time. There have been a variety of studies that have directly linked MUFA's with benefits such as insulin resistance and good cholesterol levels.

Health benefits of MUFAs:
- ✓ Better levels of HDL cholesterol
- ✓ Decrease in blood pressure
- ✓ Decreased risk of developing heart disease
- ✓ Decrease in belly fat
- ✓ Decrease in insulin resistance

Best sources of MUFAs to eat:
- ✓ Avocados and avocado oil
- ✓ Extra virgin olive oil
- ✓ Goose fat
- ✓ Lard and bacon fat
- ✓ Macadamia nut oil

POLYUNSATURATED FATS: When it comes to consuming polyunsaturated fatty acids (PUFAs), it boils most importantly down to the type. When PUFAs are heated up, they can create free radicals, which increase of inflammation and have been shown to increase the risk of developing cancer and heart disease.

PUFAs can be found in processed oils and other extremely healthy sources. Eating the correct kinds of PUFAs can give you benefits, especially when you incorporate them into your diet. They include Omega 3's and Omega 6's, which are essential to feeling great! The amount of PUFA's that you eat is extremely crucial. The ratio of omega 3 to omega 6 should be around 1:1. But most of Western diets consume a ratio of 1:30.

Health benefits of PUFAs:

When you consume a good balance of omega 3 and omega 6, you greatly reduce the risk of developing the following:

- ✓ Autoimmune disorders and other inflammatory diseases
- ✓ Heart disease
- ✓ Intake of PUFAs may even help improve symptoms of depression and help those with ADHD, which are more benefits associated on the Freestyle plan.
- ✓ Stroke

Best sources of PUFA's to eat:

- ✓ Avocado oil
- ✓ Chia seeds
- ✓ Extra virgin olive oil
- ✓ Fatty fish and fish oil
- ✓ Flaxseeds and flaxseed oil
- ✓ Nut oils
- ✓ Sesame oil
- ✓ Walnuts

TRANS FATS: You are probably questioning the author's intelligence seeing trans fats under the "good" fats category. But it does have a right to be in this section! Yes, the majority of trans fats are wildly unhealthy and can be very harmful to the human body, there *is* a type of trans fat, known as *vaccenic acid*, that is good for you! It is naturally found in foods like grass-fed meats and dairy products.

Health benefits of vaccenic acid can include:

- ✓ Decreased risk of developing diabetes and obesity
- ✓ Decreased risk of developing heart disease
- ✓ Protection against developing cancer

Best sources of healthy and natural trans fats to eat:

- ✓ Dairy fats such as butter and yogurt
- ✓ Grass-fed animal products

BAD FATS in your diet: One of the positive aspects that attract many people to the Freestyle plan is that they can consume lots of satisfying foods and healthy fats. But, lurking around the corner, there are also bad fats that you must keep an eye out for. You want to get rid of and eliminate these pesky guys, so you don't damage your bodily health. One of the key things to remember is that the quality of the food genuinely matters.

PROCESSED TRANS AND POLYUNSATURATED FATS: Processed trans fats are a common type of fat that many of you are familiar with. They have the capability of being wildly detrimental to your overall physical wellbeing. Artificial trans fats are created during the production of food, which occurs when polyunsaturated fats are processed. Therefore, it's important to only choose PUFAs that are unprocessed that are not overheated or altered in any way. Not The processing of PUFAs creates free radicals that are harmful when consumed and they are made from oils that contain genetically modified seeds.

Risks of consuming trans fats include:
- ✓ Bad for the health of your gut
- ✓ Increased risk of developing cancer
- ✓ Increased risk of developing heart disease
- ✓ Lead cause of inflammatory health issues
- ✓ Decrease in the good HDL cholesterol and increase of bad LDL cholesterol

Examples of trans fats to *eliminate*:
- ✓ Hydrogenated and partially hydrogenated oils that are in processed products like cookies, crackers, margarine, and fast food.
- ✓ Processed vegetable oils like cottonseed, sunflower, safflower, soybean, and canola oils

MAIN TAKEAWAYS: Don't fear saturated fats, but instead opt for fats that are as unprocessed as possible. If you avoid fats and oils found in processed, packaged foods that were made in a factory, you will be golden and stay on the right track to healthy success. Keep in mind that the entire purpose of the Freestyle plan is to improve your health, which includes not only maintaining the proper fat, protein, and carb ratio but picking out sources of food that promote your wellbeing and overall physical health!

INSTANT POT 101

REVOLUTIONARY...

The Instant Pot is the brand name for a programmable countertop multi-cooker. Specifically, the device itself is a single countertop appliance that can perform multiple functions. The instant pot can replace the following:

- ✓ Slow Cooker
- ✓ Pressure Cooker
- ✓ Rice Cooker
- ✓ Steamer
- ✓ Sauté/Browning Pan
- ✓ Yogurt Maker
- ✓ Warming Pan

Did you forget to thaw out something for dinner? No problem—the Instant Pot can handle it! The instant pot can cook baked potatoes in minutes and come out so fluffy on the inside too – tasty! Also, it can cook veggies in about five minutes while also preserving their nutrients. It's also a slow cooker too. Did you catch that—it's a slow cooker that doesn't boil over! When it's finished slow cooking, it goes to the warm setting. Your food doesn't continue to cook, instead the instant pot keeps it warm! This single appliance has changed the way I cook! Most days, I use the Slow Cooker or Instant Pot features. Because of this, I spend less time in the kitchen and more time doing the things I love. My grocery basket is now filled with vegetables because the instant pot perfectly cooks them while not destroying any of their nutrients.

Once a week, I cook up a batch of hardboiled eggs for a quick breakfast when I must take my grandchildren to school early in the morning. The sauté/browning feature means that I can sauté veggies and brown meat in a single pot before setting the slow cooker. I occasionally toss things in the pot and set it to the warming feature. It will warm up my food and keep it warm for hours! You can put frozen soup into the pot in the morning, set it on Warm, and have perfectly heated soup for dinner ten hours later. This single appliance has made cooking faster and more convenient (Even my husband has taken to using it!). I love that I can cook steel-cut oats for breakfast in a fraction of the time it would take on the stovetop, make rice to go with a last-minute stir-fry is in minutes, and slow-cook a stew. In fact, it's even taken the place of my slow cooker, which has since been moved out of the kitchen.

Is the Instant Pot Safe?

You might be wondering why I would want an instant pot. Don't they occasionally explode and leave sweet potatoes on the ceiling? Well, this is not your grandmother's instant pot! Modern instant pots, or pressure cookers, have several safety features that are electronically controlled. It is impossible to open the lid of one until the pressure has been released either naturally or manually—so burning hazards are minimized! Rest assured, modern day electric pressure cookers like the Instant Pot are quiet, safe and easy to use. They have 10 UL Certified proven safety mechanisms to prevent most potential issues. This means that they are very safe to use in your kitchen provided you use your common sense—for example, be careful with water spillages and keep your instant pot away from children, pets and vulnerable people.

Don't pre-heat the cooker!

I got into the habit of preheating the base of the pressure cooker on a low flame to give me time to slice onions or peel garlic cloves while the cooker was pre-heating. But, on induction, I kept getting burned olive oil and charred onions. Don't pre-heat your cooker on induction because the cooking surface is hot and ready to sauté in 15 seconds!

Don't bring the cooker to pressure on high heat!

Following the old standby advice about bringing the cooker to pressure on high heat, several obvious things will happen: the cooker reaches pressure at break-neck speed (about 4 minutes), tomato sauces carbonize and bond to the base of the cooker and the food comes out disappointingly under-done.

Don't walk away from a full cooker after you've adjusted the heat!

Although the cooker may have reached the correct pressure, the sides are still at a lower temperature than the hot aluminum-disk-clad base. Walking away from the cooker once it has cooled will cause the internal pressure to quickly fall because the heat generated from the base is not enough to keep the food inside boiling and maintaining pressure and heat up the rest of the cooker or food inside of it.

Do's!

✓ **DO** bring the pressure cooker to pressure on medium heat or tack on a few minutes to the cooking time to compensate for the lower pressure cooking temperature and shorter time to pressure.

✓ **DO** hang around to make heat adjustments for the first 5 minutes of pressure for very full or very wide cookers.

✓ **DO** use the induction burner's timer feature to set the pressure cooking time so the burner turns itself off automatically when time is up!

✓ **DO** slice the aromatics first, and then turn on the induction burner just before tossing oil or aromatics to sauté.

INSTANT POT FAQS

Is the instant pot the same as a pressure cooker?

Absolutely! The Instant Pot is currently one of the most popular electric pressure cooker brands. It is a multi-functional cooker that has some extra functions compared to traditional stove-top pressure cookers – it is also incredibly faster too!

Instapot or instant pot?

Many people call the Instant Pot a pressure cooker, InstaPot, IP or IPPY. The correct name is Instant Pot but call it whatever you like. In fact, some users even name their cookers. I call mine Toby after my childhood dog. In fact, you can also buy swanky covers to put on it too.

Is it easy to cook with an instant pot?

There's a learning curve to cook with pressure cookers. But no worries! Once you're familiar with it, you will find the cooking relatively easy.

Does the instant pot really speed up the cooking process?

Cooking in any pressure cooker is almost always faster. It may not be noticeable for some foods like broccoli or shrimps. However, tender and juicy pulled pork can be done in under 90 minutes, when it usually takes 2 – 4 hours to make in the oven.

Are there disadvantages cooking in the instant pot?

One disadvantage cooking with any pressure cooker is that you can't inspect, taste or adjust the food along the way. That's why it's essential to follow recipes with accurate cooking times (like those recipes in this book).

Can I use the instant pot for pressure frying?

Please don't attempt to pressure fry in any electric pressure cookers. The splattering oil may melt the gasket. KFC uses a commercial pressure fryer (modern ones operate at 5 PSI) specially made to fry chickens. The Chicken recipes in this book is probably as close as it gets.

How to do a quick release?

After the cooking cycle ends, carefully move the venting knob from sealing position to venting position. This rapidly releases the pressure in the pressure cooker. This usually takes a few minutes. Wait until the floating valve (metal pin) completely drops before opening the lid.

How to do a natural release?

After the cooking cycle ends, wait until the floating valve (metal pin) completely drops before opening the lid. Always turn the venting knob from sealing position to venting position. This ensures all the pressure is released before opening the lid. It usually takes 10 – 25 minutes. In these recipes, you may see "15 mins Natural Release" – this means after the cooking cycle ends, wait 15 minutes before turning the venting knob to manually release the remaining pressure.

Freestyle
RECIPES

Breakfast Spinach Delight

This recipe needs 10 minutes of preparation, 20 minutes of cooking time, and will make 4 servings.

Nutrition: 200 Cal., 3g Fat, 5g Carbs, 7g Protein.
6 Smart Points.

Ingredients:

- ✓ ½ t. turmeric
- ✓ 1 pinch cayenne pepper
- ✓ 1 t. garam masala
- ✓ 1 t. ground coriander
- ✓ 1 t. ground cumin
- ✓ 4 garlic cloves – minced
- ✓ 2 yellow onion – chopped
- ✓ 1 ginger piece
- ✓ 2 Tbsp. olive oil
- ✓ 1 lb. torn spinach
- ✓ 1 lb. mustard leaves
- ✓ 1 pinch dried fenugreek leaves
- ✓ 1 pinch black pepper

How to Make

1. Turn on your Instant Pot and place it in Sauté mode. Now add the oil and heat it up.
2. When the oil is warm, add the fenugreek, pepper, cayenne pepper, turmeric, garam masala, cumin, coriander, ginger, garlic, and onion. Cook these for five minutes.
3. Afterwards, add the mustard and spinach leaves and stir for a while.
4. Add the lid to the pot and cook these ingredients on a high setting for 15 minutes.
5. Divide into bowls and serve.

Breakfast Cobbler

This recipe needs 10 minutes of preparation, 10 minutes of cooking time and will make 4 servings.

Nutrition: 154 Cal., 2g Fat, 5g Carbs, 3g Protein
5 Smart Points.

Ingredients:

- ✓ 1 apple – chopped and cored
- ✓ 1 pear – chopped
- ✓ 1 plum – chopped
- ✓ 2 Tbsp. pecans – chopped
- ✓ 2 Tbsp. sunflower seeds
- ✓ ¼ c. coconut – shredded
- ✓ 3 Tbsp. coconut oil
- ✓ ½ t. ground cinnamon
- ✓ 2 Tbsp. honey

How to Make

1. Add oil into your Instant Pot and heat it up using Sauté mode.
2. When the oil is nice and warm, add the honey, plum, pear and apple.
3. Stir these ingredients around and then cover up the pot. Cook this on Steam mode for the next ten minutes.
4. Divide the fruit mixture between your plates and then sprinkle on the coconut, pecans and sunflower seeds before serving.

French Baked Eggs

This recipe needs 5 minutes of preparation, 8 minutes of cooking time and will make 4 servings.

Nutrition: 221 Cal., 16.1g Fat, 17.2g Protein, 1.8g Net Carbs
9 Smart Points.

Ingredients

- ✓ 4 eggs
- ✓ 4 slices of favorite meat or vegetable
- ✓ 4 slices of cheese
- ✓ fresh herbs - garnish
- ✓ olive oil
- ✓ 1 c. water

How to Make

1. Add a trivet and water into your Instant Pot.
2. Prepare the ramekins by drizzling in a drop of olive oil, coating them well.
3. Add the meat and vegetables.
4. Break an egg and drop it into the ramekin and top with cheese. Leave uncovered for harder cooked eggs.
5. Place this lot into a steamer basket and Lock the lid, close the valve and press Manual / Low and 4 minutes on the timer.
6. Release the pressure manually.
7. Finally, remove the ramekins and serve.

Mashed Cauliflower

This recipe needs 1 minute to prepare, 5 minutes to cook, and will prepare enough mashed cauliflower for 4 servings.

Protein: 10.7g, Net Carbs: 7g, Fats: 19.1g, Calories: 251
11 Smart Points.

Ingredients

- ✓ Cauliflower (1 large head, cut into chunks and core removed)
- ✓ Water (1 C or 250mL)
- ✓ Butter (1 T)
- ✓ Garlic Powder (.25 TSP)
- ✓ Chives (1 handful)

What to Make

1. Prepare your cauliflower by removing the excess leaves—if necessary,
2. Add the steamer basket into your instant pot and fill it with water.
3. Add the cauliflower chunks.
4. Close the lid and manually set your instant pot to the high-pressure setting.
5. Cook for 4 minutes.
6. Perform a quick release as per your instant pot manual's guidelines.
7. Then, carefully remove the cauliflower from the instant pot and transfer it into a bowl.
8. In the bowl with the cauliflower, add the butter and any desired seasonings.
9. Mash or blend the cauliflower with an immersion blender until you reach a creamy smooth consistency.
10. Serve & enjoy!

Ham, Sausage & Bacon Quiche

This recipe needs 10 minutes of preparation, 30 minutes of cooking time and will make 4 servings.

Nutrition: 243 Cal., 3g Fat, 6g Carbs, 12g Protein
7 Smart Points.

Ingredients:

- ✓ 2 green onions – chopped
- ✓ 1/5 c. ham – chopped
- ✓ 1 c. sausage – cooked
- ✓ 4 bacon slices – cooked
- ✓ ½ c. coconut milk
- ✓ Pepper
- ✓ 6 eggs – whisked
- ✓ 1 c. water

How to Make

1. Add water to the bottom of your Instant Pot and add the steamer basket.
2. Take out a bowl and put the ham, sausage and bacon into it. Spread this into the bottom of a quiche dish.
3. In another bowl, mix the eggs together with the green onions, coconut milk and pepper. Pour this on top of your meat mixture in the dish.
4. Add the baking dish into the Instant Pot and cover.
5. Cook on a high setting for 30 minutes.
6. Slice the quiche up and serve.

Morning Frittata

This recipe needs 10 minutes of preparation, 18 minutes of cooking time, and will make 4 servings.

Nutrition: 153 Cal., 7g Fat, 5g Carbs, 15g Protein
5 Smart Points.

Ingredients:

- ✓ 6 eggs
- ✓ 4 oz. sliced sweet potatoes – sliced
- ✓ 1 chopped green bell pepper – chopped
- ✓ 1 t. tomato paste
- ✓ ¼ c. coconut milk
- ✓ 1 minced garlic cloves – minced
- ✓ ¼ c. chopped scallions – chopped
- ✓ 1 Tbsp. olive oil
- ✓ Pepper
- ✓ Salt
- ✓ 1 ½ c. water

How to Make

1. Grease a baking dish with oil and add the sweet potato fries.
2. Now take out a bowl and mix the garlic, bell pepper, scallions, pepper, salt and eggs together.
3. Take out a second bowl and mix the tomato paste and coconut milk together.
4. Pour the milk mixture over the egg mixture and stir well. When everything is well combined, pour this on top of your sweet potato fries.
5. Add water to your Instant Pot and place a steamer basket inside. Add your baking dish with the eggs inside the steamer basket.
6. Cover the Instant Pot and cook on a high setting for 18 minutes.
7. Finally, slice up the frittata and enjoy.

Bacon Ranch Sweet Potatoes

This recipe needs 3 minutes of preparation, 12 minutes of cooking time and will make 6 servings.

Nutrition: 227 Cal., 12.3g Fat, 5.3g Protein, 24.5g Net Carbs. **11 Smart Points.**

Ingredients

- ✓ 2lb sweet potatoes - scrubbed and cubed.
- ✓ 3 bacon strips - cut
- ✓ 2 t. dried parsley
- ✓ 1 t. each kosher salt and garlic powder
- ✓ 1/3 c. ranch dressing
- ✓ 2T water

How to Make

1. Put potatoes, bacon, garlic powder, parsley, salt, and water in Instant Pot and stir.
2. Lock lid, close valve, and hit Manual/ High and 7 minutes on the timer.
3. Let pressure vent naturally for 3 - 5 minutes and then use quick-release.
4. Top with ranch dressing and serve.

Eggs De Provence

This recipe needs 10 minutes of preparation, 30 minutes of cooking time and will make 6 servings.

Nutrition: 220 Cal., 16.3g Fat, 14.6g Protein, 4g Net Carbs **11 Smart Points.**

Ingredients

- ✓ 6 eggs
- ✓ 1 c. cooked ham
- ✓ 1 small onion - chopped
- ✓ 1 c cheddar cheese
- ✓ Heavy cream (.5 c)
- ✓ Seal salt (to taste)
- ✓ Ground black pepper (to taste)
- ✓ 1 c. water

How to Make

1. Add water to your Instant Pot and add a trivet.
2. In a medium bowl, whisk the eggs and heavy cream.
3. Add the rest of the ingredients before mixing everything thoroughly.
4. Add the mixture to the heatproof dish, cover, and place it into your Instant Pot.
5. Lock the lid, close the valve, and hit Manual/ High for 20 minutes on a timer.
6. Let the pressure vent naturally and serve immediately.

Loaded Sweet Potatoes

This recipe needs 5 minutes of preparation, 20 minutes of cooking time and will make 4 servings

Nutrition: 600 Cal., 35.8g Fat, 30.4g Protein, 38.9g Net Carbs. **26 Smart Points.**

Ingredients

- ✓ 3 eggs
- ✓ 1 diced orange bell pepper
- ✓ 1 lb pork sausage
- ✓ 3 sweet potatoes
- ✓ 1/4 c. onion - diced
- ✓ 1 red bell pepper - diced
- ✓ 1/2 t. each garlic powder and meat/potato seasoning
- ✓ pinch each of sea salt and pepper
- ✓ 4 c. water

How to Make

1. Add water to your Instant Pot and insert a steamer rack.
2. Place the sweet potatoes onto the rack.
3. Lock the lid, close the valve, and cook for 20 minutes.
4. In a non-stick skillet, sauté the onions for a few minutes, until soft and slightly translucent.
5. Add the sausage and let them brown slightly.
6. Sprinkle in the garlic powder, meat/potatoes seasoning and salt/pepper. Stir well.
7. Add the eggs, stirring occasionally until slightly under-done.
8. Add the peppers and sauté for about 2 minutes.
9. Take the potatoes out of the Instant Pot and allow them to cool for about 5 minutes.
10. Use a fork to lightly scrape out the inside of the potato and mix with a skillet.
11. With a slotted spoon, stuff the inside of the potato and serve.

Sweet Potato Hash

This recipe needs 10 minutes of preparation, 10 minutes of cooking time and will make 4 servings.

Nutrition: 357 Cal., 23.7g Fat, 21g Protein, 14.7g Net Carbs. **16 Smart Points.**

Ingredients

- ✓ 1/2-sausage (pork)
- ✓ 1 large sweet potato – cubed
- ✓ Garlic (2 cloves minced)
- ✓ 1 bell pepper - seeded and diced
- ✓ 1 T Italian seasoning
- ✓ Ground black pepper (to taste)
- ✓ Sea salt (to taste)
- ✓ 2 c. water
- ✓ 1 small onion chopped
- ✓ Half a dozen eggs

How to Make

1. In a medium bowl, whisk the eggs, salt/pepper and Italian seasoning together.
2. Press the Sauté button on your Instant Pot and add the sausage, sweet potato, garlic, onion and pepper for 3–5 minutes.
3. Spoon the mixture into a greased glass dish and add the eggs.
4. Place a trivet inside your Instant Pot and add some water.
5. Place the dish with the egg mixture onto the trivet.
6. Lock the lid, close the valve, and hit Manual and 20 minutes on the timer.
7. Remove the dish and let it cool for 5–10 minutes to allow the eggs to set.
8. Slice and serve.

Hard-Boiled Eggs

This recipe needs 2 minutes of preparation, 7 minutes of cooking time and will make 4 servings.

Nutrition: 63 Cal., 4.4g Fat, 5.6g Protein, 0.4g Net Carbs.
2 Smart Points.

Ingredients

- ✓ 4 eggs
- ✓ 1/4 t. paprika
- ✓ salt to taste
- ✓ 1 c. water

How to Make

1. Add some water to your Instant Pot and insert a steamer basket inside of it.
2. Place the eggs into the basket and add in the paprika.
3. Lock the lid, close the valve and hit Manual / High for 7 minutes on the timer.
4. Perform the quick-release method and let the eggs cool slightly before serving.
5. Season with salt or paprika as desired.

Korean Style Steamed Eggs

This recipe needs 5 minutes of preparation, 5 minutes of cooking time and will make 1 servings.

Nutrition: 72 Cal., 5g Fat, 6.3g Protein, 0.5g Net Carbs.
3 Smart Points.

Ingredients

- ✓ 1 large egg
- ✓ 1 t. scallions - chopped
- ✓ pinch each of sesame seeds, garlic powder, salt, and pepper
- ✓ 1/3 c. water
- ✓ 1 c. water

How to Make

1. Pour 1 c. of water into your Instant Pot and place a trivet inside.
2. In a small bowl, mix the egg and 1/3 c. water.
3. Strain the mixture over a fine-mesh strainer into a heat-proof bowl.
4. Add the remaining ingredients, mix well and set aside.
5. Place the bowl with the egg mixture onto the trivet or steamer.
6. Lock the lid, close the valve and hit Manual / High for 5 minutes on the timer.
7. Perform the quick-release method and serve.

Egg Cups on The Go

Prep time: 10 minutes. Cooking time: 10 minutes
Yields: 4 servings.

Nutrition: 301 Cal., 21 g Fat, 13 g Prot., 4 g Net Carbs.
14 Smart Points

Ingredients

- ✓ 2 tbsp. cilantro
- ✓ Pepper and salt
- ✓ ¼ C. half and half
- ✓ ½ C. shredded sharp cheddar cheese
- ✓ 1 C. diced veggies, such as tomatoes, mushrooms bell peppers, onions
- ✓ 4 eggs
- ✓ ½ C. shredded cheese for the top

How to make

1. In a bowl, combine the cilantro, pepper, salt, half & half, cheese, veggies and eggs together.
2. Pour the mixture into 4 jars. Put on the lid, not too tightly.
3. Pour 2 cups of water into your instant pot and place a trivet on top.
4. Put the egg jars on the trivet.
5. Cook on HIGH for 5 minutes.
6. Quickly release the pressure.
7. Top the jars with ½ cup of cheese.
8. Broil for 2-3 minutes in an oven until the cheese melts and is lightly browned.
9. Serve and enjoy.

Breakfast Casserole

Prep time: 10 minutes. Cooking time: 25 minutes
Yields: 6 servings.

Nutrition: 280 Cal., 9 g Fat, 25 g Prot., 7 g Net Carbs.
9 Smart Points.

Ingredients

- ✓ 1 ½ C. cooked breakfast sausage
- ✓ 2/3 C. peeled and grated sweet potato
- ✓ 8 eggs
- ✓ 1 C. chopped kale
- ✓ 2 tsp. minced garlic cloves
- ✓ 1 1/3 C. sliced leek
- ✓ 1 ½ C. water

How to make

1. Press the sauté button on your instant pot and melt the coconut oil.
2. Add the kale, garlic, and leeks inside the pot, sautéing till softened.
3. Remove the veggies and clean out the inner pot.
4. Combine the sautéed veggies, sausage, sweet potato and eggs in a bowl. Pour into a greased bowl or pan.
5. Pour the water into the pot and place a trivet on top. Add the filled bowl carefully onto the trivet.
6. Set to cook for 25 minutes on MANUAL. Perform a quick release method to release the pressure.
7. Cut into slices and devour!

Coconut Yogurt

Prep time: 5 minutes. Cooking time: 8 hours
Yields: 6-8 servings.

Nutrition: 176 Cal., 18 g Fat, 11 g Prot., 3 g Net Carbs.
9 Smart Points.

Ingredients
- ✓ 1 tbsp. raw honey or maple syrup
- ✓ 1 tbsp. gelatin
- ✓ 4 probiotic capsules
- ✓ 3 14-ounce cans of chilled coconut milk

How to make
1. With a spoon, take the solid cream off the top of the cans of coconut milk and add it inside the instant pot.
2. Close and press the YOGURT function. Adjust until it says BOIL.
3. When the timer sounds, remove and let cool. With a thermometer, wait till the temperature reads 100 degrees.
4. Open probiotic capsules and whisk in coconut cream.
5. Place the bowl back into the instant pot and set the timer for 8 hours.
6. Pour the mixture into a blender and add the gelatin gradually as you blend.
7. Then, add additional flavorings of your choice (Honey, maple syrup, vanilla, etc.)
8. Chill for a few hours to let cool and thicken.

Sunday Pot Roast

Prep time: 5 minutes. Cooking time: 8 hours
Yields: 1 serving.

Nutrition: 200 Cal., 18 g Fat, 11 g Prot., 3 g Net Carbs.
10 Smart Points.

Ingredients
- ✓ Pepper and salt
- ✓ Cubed potatoes (1 pound)
- ✓ Carrots (3 large)
- ✓ Fat-free beef broth (1.5 c)
- ✓ Worcestershire sauce (3 tablespoons)
- ✓ Chopped onion (1 large)
- ✓ Onion soup mix (1 packets)
- ✓ Olive oil (1 tablespoon)
- ✓ Beef chuck roast (3 pounds)

How to make
1. Rub the meat all over with the pepper and salt.
2. In a bowl mix together the onion soup mix, broth, Worcestershire sauce together.
3. Turn your instant pot to the sauté setting. Once the pot has heated up, add in the oil. Place the meat in the pot and sear on all its sides, around one to two minutes on each side.
4. Add the carrots, potatoes and onions. Pour the sauce over everything.
5. Switch the pot off the sauté mode. Place the lid on the pot and seal it into place. Turn the pot to the manual setting and set it for 70 minutes at high pressure.
6. Once the cooking time is up, allow the pressure to release for ten minutes naturally, and then quick release the rest of the pressure.
7. Remove the lid and take the pot roast out. You can shred or slice the roast.
8. Serve the roast with the vegetables and enjoy.

Loaded Cauliflower Soup

Prep time: 15 minutes - Cooking time: 20 minutes
Yields: 4 servings.

Nutrition: 312 Cal., 28 g Fat, 14 g Prot., 4 g Net Carbs.
16 Smart Points.

Ingredients
- ✓ ½ C. half & half
- ✓ 1 C. grated sharp cheddar cheese
- ✓ 4 ounces cream cheese
- ✓ 1 tsp. salt
- ✓ 1 tsp. garlic powder
- ✓ 3 C. chicken stock
- ✓ 1 head cauliflower
- ✓ 2 tbsp. Butter
- ✓ ½ chopped onion

Toppings
- ✓ Green onions
- ✓ 8-10 strips bacon
- ✓ Sour cream
- ✓ Grated sharp cheddar cheese

How to make
1. Peel your onion and chop it into pieces.
2. Cut off the leaves of the cauliflower and chop it into pieces.
3. Press the SAUTE button on your instant pot. Melt the butter and place the onions inside, sautéing for 2-3 minutes.
4. Add the cauliflower, salt, garlic powder and chicken stock.
5. Lock the lid and press MANUAL. Cook on HIGH for 5 minutes.
6. Perform a quick release method.
7. While the soup cooks, cook the bacon.
8. Check to see if the cauliflower is tender. Then push KEEP WARM on the pot.
9. With an immersion blender, puree the soup. Add more stock to adjust the thickness if you choose.
10. Pour in the cream cheese and grated cheese, stirring to combine.
11. Then add in half & half, and season with pepper and salt to achieve desired taste.
12. Serve the soup hot along with green onion, crumbled bacon, sour cream and grated cheese.

Jamaican Pork Roast

Prep time: 5 minutes - Cooking time: 45 minutes
Yields: 4 servings.

Nutrition: 308 Cal., 18 g Fat, 31 g Prot., 5 g Net Carbs.
11 Smart Points.

Ingredients
- ✓ ½ C. beef stock
- ✓ 1 tbsp. olive oil
- ✓ ¼ C. Jamaican Jerk spice blend
- ✓ 4 pounds pork shoulder

How to make
1. Rub down the roast with olive oil and the spice blend.
2. Push the SAUTE button on your instant pot. Brown the meat on all sides.
3. Pour in the beef broth.
4. Seal the lid. Press MANUAL and cook on HIGH for 45 minutes.
5. Perform the quick release method.
6. Shred the pork and serve.

Juicy Instant Pot Chicken

Prep time: 10 minutes - Cooking time: 25 minutes
Yields: 8 servings.

Nutrition: 298 Cal., 14 g Fat, 29 g Prot., 2 g Net Carbs.
10 Smart Points.

Ingredients

- ✓ 6 minced cloves garlic
- ✓ ½ tsp. salt
- ✓ 2 tbsp. lemon juice
- ✓ ¼ tsp. pepper
- ✓ 1 tsp. dried thyme
- ✓ 1 ½ C. organic chicken broth
- ✓ 1 tsp. paprika
- ✓ 1 tbsp. coconut oil
- ✓ 4 pounds chicken

How to make

1. Mix together the pepper, salt, thyme and paprika. Rub the seasoning onto the chicken.
2. Warm up the oil inside your instant pot.
3. Place the chicken into the pot, breast side down, cooking 6-7 minutes.
4. Flip over the chicken and pour in the broth and add the garlic cloves and lemon juice.
5. Lock the lid and cook on HIGH for 25 minutes.
6. Perform the natural release method.
7. Remove the chicken and allow it to cool for 5 minutes before attempting to cut.

Keto Meatballs

Prep time: 15 minutes - Cooking time: 10 minutes
Yields: 6-8 servings.

Nutrition: 328 Cal., 21 g Fat, 26 g Prot., 5 g Net Carbs.
13 Smart Points.

Ingredients

- ✓ 1/3 C. warm water
- ✓ ¼ tsp. dried oregano
- ✓ 1 tsp. dried onion flakes
- ✓ ¼ tsp. garlic powder
- ✓ ¼ tsp. pepper
- ✓ 1 tsp. salt
- ✓ 2 eggs
- ✓ ½ C. almond flour
- ✓ ¾ C. grated parmesan cheese
- ✓ 2 tbsp. chopped parsley
- ✓ 1 ½ pounds ground beef

To Cook

- ✓ 1 tsp. olive oil
- ✓ 3 C. keto marinara sauce

How to make

1. In a bowl, mix all the meatball components with your hands.
2. Form the mixture into 2" balls.
3. With the olive oil, coat your instant pot.
4. Brown the meatballs in a skillet.
5. Layer the meatballs and marinara into your instant pot.
6. Set to MANUAL and push LOW to cook for 10 minutes.
7. Perform a quick release method.
8. Serve with zoodles!

Cauliflower Mashed Potatoes

Prep time: 10 minutes - Cooking time: 5 minutes
Yields: 6 servings.

Nutrition: 179 Cal., 12 g Fat, 8 g Prot., 1 g Net Carbs.
8 Smart Points.

Ingredients:

- ✓ Pepper and salt
- ✓ Garlic powder
- ✓ 1 C. water
- ✓ 1 head cauliflower

How to make

1. Core the cauliflower and chop it into chunks.
2. Place a trivet into the instant pot. Pour in the water and add the cauliflower to the trivet.
3. Close the lid.
4. Cook on MANUAL for 3-5 minutes.
5. Perform a quick release method.
6. Take out the cauliflower and empty the pot.
7. With an immersion blender, puree till you reach a desired consistency.

Broccoli Cheese Soup

Prep time: 10 minutes - Cooking time: 5 minutes
Yields: 4 servings.

Nutrition: 329 Cal., 31 g Fat, 19 g Prot., 4 g Net Carbs.
17 Smart Points.

Ingredients

- ✓ 1 tsp. pepper and salt
- ✓ 2 C. shredded sharp cheddar cheese
- ✓ 1 C. heavy cream
- ✓ 1 C. shredded carrots
- ✓ ¼ tsp. garlic powder
- ✓ 1 bunch broccoli
- ✓ 4 C. chicken stock
- ✓ 1 tbsp. onion powder

How to make

1. Turn on your instant pot to SAUTE mode.
2. Place the butter inside the pot and melt.
3. Pour in the pepper, salt, onion powder, garlic powder, chicken stock, carrots and broccoli into the instant pot.
4. Set to cook on HIGH for 5 minutes.
5. Perform a quick release method.
6. Mix in the heavy cream and cheddar cheese.
7. Serve and enjoy!

Chicken Tikka Masala

Prep time: 15 minutes - Cooking time: 10 minutes
Yields: 6 servings.

Nutrition: 394 Cal., 22 g Fat, 18 g Prot., 4 g Net Carbs.
16 Smart Points.

5 points

Ingredients

Chicken Marinade:
- ✓ ¼ tsp. ginger
- ✓ 1 tsp. pepper
- ✓ 1 tbsp. lemon juice
- ✓ 1 tbsp. garam masala
- ✓ 1 C. 2% plain Greek yogurt
- ✓ 1-pound boneless skinless chicken breast

Sauce

- ✓ 1 C. heavy whipping cream
- ✓ ¼ tsp. cayenne pepper
- ✓ ½ tsp. salt
- ✓ ½ tsp. turmeric
- ✓ ½ tsp. paprika
- ✓ 4 tsp. garam masala
- ✓ 5 cloves minced garlic
- ✓ 15-ounce can tomato sauce

How to make

1. Mix the chicken marinade components together. Place the chunks of chicken into the marinade to coat. Allow to sit in a fridge for at least 60 minutes.
2. Press the SAUTE mode on your instant pot. Add the chunks of chicken and sauté for 5 minutes till cooked on all sides.
3. Set the instant pot to HIGH. Pour in all the sauce components into the pot and combine well
4. Cover the lid. Push MANUAL and let cook for 10 minutes. Perform a quick release method.
5. Push SAUTE again. Once the pot has warmed, add in the cream, combining well. Allow the contents of the recipe to simmer.
6. Serve on top of the rice. Top with cilantro if desired. Enjoy!

Boneless Pork Chops

Prep time: 10 minutes - Cooking time: 5 minutes
Yields: 4-6 servings.

Nutrition: 288 Cal., 19 g Fat, 24 g Prot., 6 g Net Carbs.
12 Smart Points.

Ingredients

- ✓ 1 C. water
- ✓ 1 package ranch mix
- ✓ 1 stick butter
- ✓ 4-6 boneless pork chops
- ✓ 1 tbsp. coconut oil

How to make

1. Put the pork chops inside your instant pot along with the coconut oil.
2. Push the SAUTE button and brown all the sides.
3. Put the butter on top of the chops and sprinkle with ranch mix.
4. Pour the water over the pork chops.
5. Put on the lid.
6. Push MANUAL and set to cook for 5 minutes.
7. Allow the pressure to release naturally.
8. Serve with buttery sauce over the top of the pork chops when serving.

Low-Carb Green Chili Pork Taco Bowl

Prep time: 10 minutes - Cooking time: 45 minutes
Yields: 4-6 servings.

Nutrition: 405 Cal., 27 g Fat, 34 g Prot., 3 g Net Carbs.
16 Smart Points.

Ingredients
- ✓ 16 ounces of green Chile salsa
- ✓ 1 tbsp. olive oil
- ✓ 1 tsp. pepper and salt
- ✓ 2 tsp. garlic powder
- ✓ 2 tsp. cumin
- ✓ 2 pounds pork sirloin

How to make
1. Trim the pork and cut it into slices against the grain.
2. Mix the pepper, salt, garlic powder and cumin together and then rub them onto the pork.
3. Press the SAUTE mode on your instant pot and brown the pork on all sides.
4. Pour in the green Chile salsa.
5. Lock the lid and push MANUAL to cook on HIGH for 45 minutes.
6. Serve with cauliflower rice.

Crack Chicken

Prep time: 5 minutes - Cooking time: 25 minutes
Yields: 4 servings.

Nutrition: 391 Cal., 23 g Fat, 29 g Prot., 2 g Net Carbs.
15 Smart Points.

Ingredients
- ✓ 4 ounces cheddar cheese
- ✓ 3 tbsp. cornstarch
- ✓ 1 C. water
- ✓ 8 ounces cream cheese
- ✓ 1 packet ranch seasoning
- ✓ 2 pounds boneless chicken breast
- ✓ 6-8 cooked bacon

How to make
1. Put the chicken into the instant pot along with the cream cheese.
2. Sprinkle the ranch seasoning over the chicken and add the water.
3. Set to MANUAL to cook on HIGH for 25 minutes.
4. Perform a quick release method.
5. Take out the chicken and shred into pieces.
6. Set the instant pot to LOW and pour in the cornstarch.
7. Add the cheese and shredded chicken to the cornstarch.
8. Mix in the bacon and devour!

Pork Carnitas

Prep time: 20 minutes - Cooking time: 50 minutes
Yields: 6-8 servings.

Nutrition: 374 Cal., 19 g Fat, 27 g Prot., 5 g Net Carbs.
14 Smart Points.

Ingredients

- ½ tsp. garlic powder
- ¼ tsp. dry adobo sauce
- 2 bay leaves
- 2-3 chipotle peppers in adobo sauce
- ¾ C. reduced-sodium chicken broth
- ¼ tsp. dried oregano
- ½ tsp. sazon
- 1 ½ tsp. cumin
- Pepper
- 2 tsp. salt
- 2 ½ pounds boneless pork shoulder blade roast

How to make

1. With the pepper and salt, season your pork shoulder.
2. Brown all the sides of the pork in a skillet for 5 minutes.
3. Take off the heat and let cool.
4. Cut a 1" insert into the meat and place the garlic slivers inside.
5. Season the pork shoulder with garlic powder, adobo, oregano, sazon and cumin.
6. Pour the broth into the instant pot and set to HIGH to cook for 50 minutes.
7. Perform a natural release method.
8. Shred the pork with two forks.
9. Combine with cooking juices. Take out bay leaves and enjoy.

Beef Pho

Prep Time: 6 min. Cooking Time: 60 min.
Yields: 8 Servings.

Nutrition: Cal. 571, 70 g Prot., 22.3 g Fat, 18.6 g Net Carbs.
17 Smart Points.

Ingredients

- 2 whole star anise
- 1 t. black peppercorns
- 6 whole cloves
- 1 t. Coriander seeds
- 1 cinnamon stick
- 1 large diced onion
- 1 tsp avocado oil/tallow
- 2 pieces - thumb-sized gender nights
- 2 lb. beef shank
- 2 lb. oxtails
- 1 tbsp. coconut sugar
- 1 t. Sea salt
- 2 tbsp. fish sauce
- 1 tbsp. Apple cider vinegar
- ¾ lb. flank steak - thinly sliced
- Rice noodles, tapioca noodles, or favorite veggie noodles
- 1 bunch Thai mint, basil, or cilantro
- Bean sprouts or spirally sliced daikons
- 1 sliced jalapeno
- Sriracha

How to Make

1. Prepare the Instant Pot using the sauté function.
2. Add the star anise, cinnamon stick, peppercorns, coriander seeds and cloves. Toast for 5 minutes.
3. Fold in the tallow, ginger and onion. Sauté for six minutes. Do not stir.
4. Then, add the spices to the pot along with the beef shank, oxtail, vinegar, coconut sugar and salt.
5. Empty 8 cups of water into the pot, just below the max line.
6. Use the high-pressure setting for 50 minutes or the meat/stew function.
7. Natural release the pressure and wait 20 minutes. Then do a quick release.
8. Use a strainer for the broth, remove all the meat, and set it to the side. Skim off the fat.
9. Stir in extra salt, fish sauce or coconut sugar to your liking. Toss the beef back to the Instant Pot to warm up.
10. Fold in the noodles of choice, flank steak, jalapenos and other seasonings to your liking.

Cauliflower Bacon & Cheese Soup

Prep Time: 25 min. Cooking Time: 33 min. Yields: 6 Servings.

Nutrition: 347 Cal., 25.6 g, Fat, 17.7 g Prot., 13.4 g Net Carbs. **16 Smart Points.**

Ingredients

- ✓ 2 minced garlic cloves
- ✓ 1 large diced onion
- ✓ 1 tbsp. olive oil
- ✓ 1 head coarsely chopped cauliflower
- ✓ 1 tbsp. onion powder
- ✓ 1 chopped green pepper- optional
- ✓ To Taste: Ground black pepper and salt
- ✓ 32 oz. container of chicken stock
- ✓ 1 tbsp. Dijon mustard
- ✓ 1 c. Half and Half
- ✓ 6 slices- diced- turkey bacon cooked
- ✓ 2 c. shredded cheddar cheese
- ✓ Hot pepper sauce- 4 dashes

How to Make

1. Select the sauté function on your Instant Pot.
2. Add the garlic, onion and olive oil. Sauté for about 3 minutes.
3. When brown, add the green pepper, cauliflower, salt, pepper and onion powder.
4. Empty the stock, close the lid, and set the timer for 15 minutes.
5. When the timer buzzes, perform a quick release method.
6. Add the Half-and-Half, cheddar cheese, turkey bacon, hot sauce and Dijon mustard.
7. Cook until bubbly for about 5 minutes.
8. Enjoy.

Chicken Curry Soup

Prep Time: 6 mins. Cooking Time: 30 mins. Yields: 6 Servings.

Nutrition: 108 Cal., 3 g Fat, 15 g Prot., 3 g Net Carbs. **3 Smart Points.**

Ingredients

- ✓ 1 ½ c. unsweetened coconut milk
- ✓ 1 lb. chicken thighs – no skin
- ✓ 3-4 crushed garlic cloves
- ✓ ½ finely diced onion
- ✓ 2-inch knob ginger – minced
- ✓ 1 c. sliced mushrooms
- ✓ 4 oz. baby spinach
- ✓ ½ t. of each:
  - o -Cayenne pepper
  - o Turmeric
- ✓ 1 t. of each:
  - o Salt
  - o Garam masala
  - o ¼ c. chopped cilantro

How to Make

1. Combine all the ingredients into the Instant Pot.
2. Set the pressure for ten minutes.
3. Perform a natural release method when done.
4. Remove and shred the thighs.
5. Add the meat to the pot.
6. Stir in the juices and meat for a minute or so.
7. Serve and enjoy!

Chicken Fajita Soup

Prep Time: 6 min. Cook Time: 30 min.
Yields: 8 Servings.

Nutrition: 346 Cal., 35.07 g Prot., 15.1 g Fat, 8.1 g Net
Carbs. **11 Smart Points.**

Ingredients

- ✓ 2 ½ lb. chicken thighs
- ✓ 1 can diced tomatoes of each:
  - ○ -Green chilis - Rotel (10 oz.)
  - ○ -Regular diced (14.5 oz.)
- ✓ 2 qt. chicken broth
- ✓ 1 t. of each:
  - ○ Salt & Black pepper
  - ○ Chili powder
  - ○ Garlic powder
- ✓ 1 pkg. seasoning blend (see below)
- ✓ ¾ chipotle powder/more chili powder

Possible Garnishes (Add the Carbs)
- ✓ Avocado
- ✓ Sour Cream
- ✓ Lime wedges
- ✓ Chopped cilantro

Note for the Blend:
You can purchase the store-bought mixture of frozen celery, peppers, and chopped onions. You can also use 2 celery stalks, ¼ of a large onion, and a chopped bag of sliced peppers.

How to Make

1. Discard all the skin and bones from the thighs.
2. Arrange all the fixings in your Instant Pot. Select the soup setting.
3. Perform a natural release method.
4. Take the chicken from the pot and chop into pieces using 2 forks.
5. Return it to the pot to reheat.
6. Serve with the desired toppings.

Chicken Korma

Prep Time: 7 min. Cooking Time: 25 min.
Yields: 6 Servings.

Nutrition: 256 Cal., 19.0 g Fat, 14 g Prot., 6 g Net Carbs.
12 Smart Points.

Ingredients

- ✓ 1 lb. chicken thighs
- ✓ 1 c. diced tomatoes
- ✓ 1 chopped onion
- ✓ ½ jalapeno/green serrano
- ✓ 5 garlic cloves
- ✓ 1 t. of each:
  - ○ Garam masala
  - ○ Salt
  - ○ Turmeric
  - ○ Minced ginger
- ✓ ½ t. of each:
  - ○ Ground coriander
  - ○ Cayenne pepper
  - ○ Ground cumin
- ✓ ½ c. water

Ingredients for the Finish
- ✓ ½ c. unsweetened coconut milk
- ✓ 1 t. garam masala
- ✓ ¼ c. chopped cilantro

How to Make

1. Combine all the veggies and spices. Add them to the Instant Pot.
2. Add the chicken and set the timer for 10 minutes (high pressure).
3. Perform a natural release method.
4. Remove the chicken and dice it into pieces.
5. Pour in the garam masala and coconut milk along with the chicken in the pot.
6. Garnish and serve.

Chicken Mushroom Soup

Prep Time: 6 min. Cooking Time: 25 min.

Yields: 4 Servings. Nutrition: 289 Cal., 15 g Fat, 30 g Prot., 9 g Net Carbs. **10 Smart Points.**

Ingredients

- ✓ 3 minced garlic cloves
- ✓ 1 thinly sliced onion
- ✓ 1 chopped yellow squash
- ✓ 2 c. mushrooms - chopped
- ✓ 1 lb. chicken breasts – remove bones and skin
- ✓ 2 ½ c. chicken stock
- ✓ Pepper & Salt
- ✓ 1 t. Poultry/Italian Seasoning

Optional: ½ c. heavy whipping cream

How to Make

1. Toss everything into your Instant Pot and cook for 15 minutes under high pressure.
2. Perform a natural release for 10 minutes, then quick release.
3. Remove the chicken and roughly puree the veggies in an immersion blender.
4. Shred the chicken and add it back into the pot.
5. Add the cream, stir, and serve.

Chicken Pot Pie Soup

Prep Time: 15 min. Cooking Time: 45 min
Yields: 6 Servings.

Nutrition: 432 Cal., 20.5 g Prot., 35.1 g Fat, 3.5 g Net Carbs. **21 Smart Points.**

Ingredients

- ✓ 2 tbsp. butter
- ✓ 1 lb. – 1 ½ lb. (thawed) skinless – boneless chicken breasts
- ✓ ¼ of a small diced onion
- ✓ ½ c. mixed veggies
- ✓ 3 c. chicken broth
- ✓ ¼ t. of each
  - ○ Black pepper
  - ○ Pink salt
- ✓ 2 minced cloves of garlic
- ✓ 1 ¾ c. heavy whipping cream
- ✓ 1 oz. cream cheese
- ✓ ¼ t. rosemary
- ✓ 1 t. poultry seasoning
- ✓ Pinch of thyme
- ✓ ½ t. xanthan gum

How to Make

1. Melt the butter in the Instant Pot using the sauté function.
2. Toss in the mixed veggies and onion. Cook for a 2 minutes until translucent.
3. Add this into a bowl and set it to the side.
4. Pour in ½ c. of the broth to deglaze the cooker. Toss in the chicken along with the spices.
5. Close the top and select the poultry setting (15 minutes).
6. Perform natural release method for 6 minutes and then perform a quick release to release the rest of the pressure.
7. Shred the chicken and add the rest of the broth, chicken, cream cheese, veggies and whipping cream into the pot.
8. Switch to the warm cycle and add the xanthan gum. Stir and sauté for about 10 minutes. Serve when ready.

Ham & Bean Soup

Prep Time: 12 min. Cooking Time: 55min.
Yields: 6 Servings.

Nutrition: 269 Cal., 21 g Prot., 14 g Fat, 13 g Net Carbs.
10 Smart Points.

Ingredients
- 1 c. of each:
  - Chopped onion
  - Dried black soybeans – after soaking yields = 2 c. beans
  - Chopped celery
- 1 t. of each:
  - Dried oregano
  - Cajun seasoning
  - Salt –½ t.
  - Liquid smoke
  - Louisiana Hot Sauce
- 4 minced garlic cloves
- 2 t. all-purpose seasoning
- 2 smoked ham hocks
- 2 c. of each:
  - Water
  - Chopped ham

How to Make
1. Add all the fixings to your Instant Pot and choose the bean/chili function (30 min. high-pressure).
2. Perform a natural release for 10 minutes, and quick release the rest of the pressure.
3. Trash the bone and add the meat back into the soup.
4. Roughly puree some of the soup with an immersion blender.
5. Enjoy piping hot with some hot sauce on the side.

Hot & Sour Soup

Prep Time: 15 min. Cooking Time: 10 min.
Yields: 8 Servings.

Nutrition: 158 Cal., 5 g Fat, 20 g Prot., 5 g Net Carbs.
4 Smart Points.

Ingredients
- 1 lb. thinly sliced pork tenderloin
- 5 c. low-sodium chicken broth
- 1 tbsp. Chinese black vinegar/white vinegar
- 2 tbsp. Chinese rice vinegar/white vinegar
- 3 tbsp. soy sauce/coconut aminos
- 1 c. dried 'woodear' mushrooms
- ½ t. xanthan gum
- 2 t. pepper
- 1 t. salt
- 3 tbsp. water

Ingredients After Soup is Cooked
- 4 lightly beaten eggs
- 1 lb. extra-firm tofu

How to Make
1. Add all the fixings into your Instant Pot (except for the eggs and tofu).
2. Use the soup function for 10 minutes (high-pressure).
3. Perform a natural release method for 15 minutes, and then a quick release. Keep the food inside warm using the sauté function.
4. Remove the mushrooms and slice thinly—adding them back in the pot. Dice the tofu and add the eggs.
5. Stir with some chopsticks and let it sauté for a minute before serving.

Italian Sausage Kale Soup

Prep Time: 12 min. Cooking Time:10 min.
Yields: 6 Servings.

Nutrition: 400 Cal., 16 g Prot., 33 g Fat, 8 g Net Carbs.
20 Smart Points.

Ingredients
- ✓ 6 minced garlic cloves
- ✓ 1 c. diced onion
- ✓ 1 lb. hot Italian sausage
- ✓ 12 oz. frozen of each:
  - o Kale
  - o Cauliflower

Ingredients for Finishing
- ✓ ½ c. of each:
  - o Shredded parmesan cheese
  - o Heavy whipping cream

How to Make
1. Remove the sausage from the casing.
2. Prepare the Instant Pot with the sauté function.
3. Add the sausage when it's hot, breaking them apart.
4. Add the garlic, onions, frozen kale and frozen cauliflower.
5. Add 3 cups of water and secure the lid.
6. Cook on high pressure for 3 minutes.
7. Perform a natural release for 5 minutes, then quick release.
8. Add the whipping cream and mix until it is the texture you desire.
9. Empty into serving dishes and garnish with some parmesan cheese.

Jalapeno Popper Soup

Prep Time: 12 min. Cooking Time: 40 min.
Yields: 8 Servings.

Nutrition: 571 Cal., 41.2 g, Prot., Fat 40.1 g, 2.1 g Net Carbs.
24 Smart Points.

Ingredients
- ✓ ½ lb. bacon – cooked and crumbled
- ✓ 1 ½ lb. chicken breasts (boneless skinless)
- ✓ ½ c. heavy whipping cream
- ✓ 3 tbsp. butter
- ✓ ½ chopped onion
- ✓ 2 minced garlic cloves
- ✓ ½ chopped green pepper
- ✓ 2 jalapenos – seeded and chopped
- ✓ 6 oz. cream cheese
- ✓ 3 c. chicken broth
- ✓ ½ t. pepper
- ✓ 1 t. of each:
  - o Salt
  - o Cumin
- ✓ ¼ t. paprika
- ✓ ½ t. xanthan gum
- ✓ ¾ c. of each cheese:
  - o Cheddar
- ✓ Monterrey Jack

How to Make
1. Prepare the Instant Pot using the sauté function. Add in the onions, butter, jalapenos, green peppers and seasoning.
2. Sauté until translucent. Stir in the cubed chicken, broth and cream cheese.
3. Set the timer for 15 minutes - manual.
4. Perform a 5 minute natural release, when a quick release after that time.
5. Choose the sauté function and remove the chicken from the bone using two forks.
6. Add the chicken, whipping cream, both kinds of cheese and the cooked bacon. Sprinkle the xanthan gum to thicken the soup.
7. Simmer a few minutes and serve with some grated cheese, jalapenos or bacon on the top.

Kimchi Beef Stew

Prep Time: 14 min. Cooking Time: 30 min.
Yields: 6 Servings.

Nutrition: 199 Cal., 40g Prot., 20g Fat, 5.5 g Net Carbs.
8 Smart Points.

Ingredients
1 lb. beef cubes – 2-inch bits
- ✓ 2 c. Kimchi
- ✓ 1 c. of each:
    - ○ Dried Shiitake/another mushroom
    - ○ Chopped onion
- ✓ 1 tbsp. of each:
    - ○ Gochujang brown rice pepper paste
    - ○ Gochugaru Korean chili powder/Cayenne pepper
    - ○ Minced garlic
    - ○ Sesame oil
    - ○ Minced ginger
    - ○ Soy sauce/coconut aminos
- ✓ ¼ t. Splenda/favorite sweetener
- ✓ 2 c. water
- ✓ To Taste: Salt

Ingredients for Finishing
- ✓ ½ c. of each:
    - ○ Diced green onion
    - ○ Optional: Diced firm tofu

How to Make
1. Empty all the fixings into your Instant Pot. Prepare on high for 15 minutes.
2. Perform a natural release for 5 minutes, and a quick release after that to release the remaining pressure.
3. Toss in the onions and tofu. Adjust the salt and add a bit more gochugaru if desired.

Mutton Curry

Prep Time: 15 min. Cook Time: 25 min.
Yields: 4 Servings.

Nutrition: 253 Cal., 24.65 g Prot., 13.5 g Fat, 6.34 g Net Carbs. **9 Smart Points.**

Ingredients
- ✓ 3 tbsp. oil/ghee
- ✓ 1 lb. mutton bone-in (1-2-inch bits)
- ✓ 1 large (11 oz.) finely chopped onion
- ✓ Optional: 1 green chili
- ✓ ½ tbsp. minced of each:
    - ○ Ginger
    - ○ Garlic
- ✓ 1 tbsp. lemon juice
- ✓ 1 med. chopped tomato
- ✓ Garnish: Cilantro

Spices
- ✓ 2 t. coriander
- ✓ 1 t. of each:
    - ○ Cayenne/red chili powder
    - ○ Salt
    - ○ Garam masala
- ✓ ¼ t. turmeric

Whole Spices
- ✓ 6 of each:
    - ○ Cloves
    - ○ Black peppercorns
- ✓ ½ t. cumin seeds
- ✓ 1 bay leaf
- ✓ 1 (1-inch) cinnamon stick
- ✓ 2 black cardamom

How to Make
1. Use the sauté function on your Instant Pot and pour in the oil. Fold in the whole spices and sauté for 30 seconds. Stir in the onions, green chilis and garlic. Sauté four minutes.
2. Blend in the spices and chopped tomatoes, stirring for another two minutes.
3. Stir in the mutton and mix well, sautéing for another two minutes.
4. Close the lid and select the meat function for 20 minutes.
5. Perform a natural release method
6. Add the lemon juice and garnish with the mutton curry and cilantro.

No Beans Beef Chili

Prep Time: 20 min. Cooking Time: 10 min
Yields: 8 Servings.

Nutrition: Cal. 326, 23 g Prot., 17g Fat, 8 g Net Carbs.
12 Smart Points.

Ingredients

- ✓ 2 lbs. beef
- ✓ can (6 Oz.) tomato paste
- ✓ cans tomato sauce (15 oz. each)
- ✓ tbsp. cumin powder
- ✓ tbsp. chili powder
- ✓ ½ c. dried onion flakes/ 1 med. onion chopped
- ✓ 1 t. Tabasco sauce
- ✓ 1 t. garlic powder/ 2 minced cloves
- ✓ 2 t. fine ground sea salt
- ✓ 1 t. powdered/ dried oregano
- ✓ For Thinning: 1 c. chicken or beef broth

How to Make

1. Finely chop the onion. Use the sauté function on your Instant Pot to brown the beef. Blend in the Tabasco, garlic or onion flakes, cumin, salt, chili powder and oregano. Mix thoroughly.
2. Empty one cup of the broth into the burger, but do not stir.
3. Stir in the tomato sauce and paste—but do not stir.
4. Close the top and use the manual high-pressure setting for 10 minutes.
5. Perform a natural release for 10 minutes, then quick release.
6. Serve.

Szechuan Pork Soup

Prep Time: 12 min. Cooking Time: 35 min.
Yields: 6 Servings.

Nutrition: 146 Cal., 10 g Prot., 8 g Fat, 7 g Net Carbs.
6 Smart Points.

Ingredients

- ✓ 2 tbsp. of each:
  - o Black vinegar
  - o Soy sauce/coconut aminos
- ✓ 1-2 t. salt – to your liking
- ✓ 2 t. Szechuan peppers-roughly chopped
- ✓ 3-inch minced ginger
- ✓ 6 minced garlic cloves
- ✓ 2 tbsp. peanut/favorite oil
- ✓ ½ sliced onion
- ✓ 2 tbsp. Chinese fermented broad bean paste - doban jiang paste
- ✓ 1 lb. pork shoulders – in chunks
- ✓ 3 c. water

Ingredients for the Finish

- • ¼ c. cilantro
- • 3-4 c. chopped bok choy- Chinese cabbage

How to Make

1. Program the Instant Pot to the sauté mode and add the oil.
2. When heated, toss in the garlic and ginger – sautéing for a minute or two.
3. Toss in the remainder of the fixings (except for the cilantro and bok choy) and mix well.
4. Set the pot on the high-pressure setting for 20 minutes.
5. Perform a natural release for 10 minutes.
6. Garnish as desired and enjoy!

Taco Soup

Prep Time: 10 min. Cooking Time: 10 min.
Yields: 8 Servings.

Nutrition: 386 Cal., 27 g Prot., 28 g Fat, 7 g Net Carbs.
17 Smart Points.

Ingredients
- ✓ 2 lb. ground beef
- ✓ 2 t. cumin
- ✓ 2 tbsp. chili powder
- ✓ 4 minced garlic cloves
- ✓ Optional: 1 tbsp. onion flakes
- ✓ 1 can (20 oz.) Rotel diced tomatoes with chilis
- ✓ 1 container (32 oz.) beef broth
- ✓ 1 pkg. (8 oz.) cream cheese
- ✓ ½ c. heavy cream
- ✓ To Taste: Salt and pepper

Optional Garnishes
- ✓ Sour cream
- ✓ Sliced black olives
- ✓ Sliced jalapeno peppers
- ✓ Shredded cheddar cheese

How to Make
1. Program your Instant Pot to the sauté function and add the diced tomatoes, onion flakes, cumin, chili powder, garlic, pepper and salt.
2. Secure the lid and set the pot on the soup function for 5 minutes.
3. Perform a natural release for 10 minutes and quick release the rest of the pressure.
4. Add the whipping cream and cream cheese. Stir.
5. Serve when hot and add the desired toppings.

Texas Chili

Prep Time: 15 min. Cooking Time: 15 min.
Yields: 4 Servings.

Nutrition: 395 Cal., 30 g Prot., 24 g Fat, 9 g Net Carbs.
16 Smart Points.

Ingredients
- ✓ 1 c. chopped onion
- ✓ 1 tbsp. of each:
  - ○ Oil
  - ○ Minced garlic
- ✓ 1 lb. ground beef
- ✓ 1 c. (canned) fire-roasted diced tomatoes
- ✓ 1 tbsp. chopped chipotle chilies in adobo sauce (canned)
- ✓ ½ c. water
- ✓ 2 corn tortillas

Ingredients for the Spice Mixture
- ✓ 1 t. dried oregano
- ✓ 2 t. of each:
  - ○ Salt
  - ○ -Ground cumin
- ✓ 3 t. Mexican red chili powder – not Cayenne

How to Make
1. Use the Instant Pot sauté function to warm the oil. Toss in the garlic and onion—stirring for approximately 30 seconds. Toss in the beef as you break it apart.
2. Blend the chipotle chili, canned tomatoes and tortillas until smooth.
3. Combine the spices in a small dish. Add to the beef and simmer for about 30 seconds.
4. Stir in the tortilla mixture and tomatoes. Add about ½ c. of water into the emptied blender and pour it into the Instant Pot.
5. Secure the lid and cook for ten minutes on high pressure.
6. Perform a ten-minute natural release and a quick release to release the rest of the pressure.
7. Stir and top off with some cheese (add the carbs) and serve.

Thai Yellow Curry Soup

Prep Time: 15 min. Cooking Time: 12 min.
Yields: 6 Servings.

Nutrition: 345 Cal., 14 g Prot., 29 g Fat, 7 g Net Carbs.
17 Smart Points.

Ingredients
- ✓ 4 skinless – boneless chicken thighs
- ✓ 3 t. soy sauce/coconut aminos
- ✓ 2 t. of each:
  - o Fish sauce
  - o Thai yellow curry paste
- ✓ 1 full-fat (14.5 oz.) unsweetened coconut milk
- ✓ 2 chopped green onions
- ✓ 1 t. honey/agave nectar/another sweetener of choice
- ✓ 4 crushed garlic cloves
- ✓ 2-inch finely chopped portion minced ginger

Veggies to Add
- ✓ ½ c. grape tomato slices
- ✓ Optional: 1 can straw mushrooms
- ✓ ¼ c. chopped cilantro
- ✓ 3 chopped green onions
- ✓ 1 juiced lime

How to Make
1. Toss the main ingredients for the soup into the Instant Pot and secure the lid.
2. Program the pot using the soup function (12 min. high-pressure).
3. Perform a quick release method and shred the chicken, adding it back to the pot.
4. Chop the tomatoes in half and add the rest of the ingredients to the cooker.
5. Cook until heated and serve.

Unstuffed Cabbage Roll Soup

Prep Time: 16 min. Cooking Time: 25 min.
Yields: 9 Servings.

Nutrition: 217 Cal., 15.6 g Prot., 14.8 g Fat, 4.3 g Net Carbs.
9 Smart Points.

Ingredients
- ✓ 2 minced garlic cloves
- ✓ ½ small diced onion
- ✓ 1 ½ lb. ground beef – 80/20
- ✓ ¼ c. Bragg's Aminos
- ✓ 1 can (8oz.) tomato sauce
- ✓ 3 c. beef broth
- ✓ 3 t. Worcestershire sauce 'keto' approved/another substitute
- ✓ 1 can diced tomatoes (14 oz.)
- ✓ 1 med. chopped cabbage
- ✓ ½ t. of each:
  - o Pepper
  - o Parsley
  - o Salt

How to Make
1. Prepare your Instant Pot using the sauté function to brown the beef, garlic and onions.
2. Drain and add them back to the pot with the rest of the ingredients.
3. Program the pot using the soup function.
4. Perform a natural release method for about ten minutes, and then a quick release to release the rest of the steam.
5. Stir and serve.

White Chicken Chili

Prep Time: 5 min. Cooking Time: 20 min.
Yields: 4 Servings.

Nutrition: 204 Cal., 12 g Fat, 15 g Prot., 6 g Net Carbs.
8 Smart Points.

Ingredients

- ✓ 2 lb. chicken breasts – skinless – boneless
- ✓ 4 diced celery stalks
- ✓ 2 diced onions
- ✓ 10 minced garlic cloves
- ✓ 1-2 minced jalapeno peppers
- ✓ 1 t. of each:
    - ○ Coriander powder
    - ○ Cumin
    - ○ Oregano
- ✓ 1 tbsp. salt – to taste
- ✓ ¼ t. freshly cracked black pepper
- ✓ 1 tbsp. chili powder
- ✓ 4 c. chicken broth
- ✓ 1 pkg. frozen (1 lb.) corn
- ✓ 1 can (15 oz.) cannellini beans – rinsed

For Serving:

- ✓ Cilantro
- ✓ Hot Sauce

How to Make

1. Mix all the ingredient into your Instant Pot (except for the beans and corn).
2. Secure the lid and set the pot on high pressure for 15 minutes.
3. Perform a quick release the pressure and shred the chicken in the pot, adding the corn and cannellini beans.
4. Sauté for 5 minutes until heated. Serve.

Beef Chili

This recipe needs 5 minutes to prepare, 30 minutes to cook, and will prepare enough chili for 4 servings.

Protein: 39.1g. Net Carbs: 6.1g. Fats: 41.9g. Calories: 570.
25 Smart Points.

Ingredients

- ✓ Ground Beef (1lb)
- ✓ Onion (.5 Cup or 125mL, chopped)
- ✓ Red Pepper (1 Cup or 250mL, diced)
- ✓ Salt (.75 TSP)
- ✓ Ground Cumin (1 TSP)
- ✓ Black Beans (15oz can, rinsed)
- ✓ Garlic Powder (.25 TSP)
- ✓ Tomato Sauce (.5 cup or 125mL)
- ✓ Diced Tomatoes with Green Chilies (10oz can, drained)
- ✓ Broth (.75 C or 190mL)
- ✓ Chili Powder (.5 TSP)
- ✓ Paprika (.5 TSP)

How to Make

1. Sauté your beef in your instant pot until completely browned. Break it apart as you sauté it.
2. Cook the onions and peppers until the onion becomes translucent.
3. Add the tomatoes, spices, broth and beans.
4. Cover and cook by manually setting the pot to high pressure for 20 minutes.
5. Perform the natural release method.
6. Serve and enjoy.

Chicken Chili Verde

This recipe needs 10 minutes to prepare, 30 minutes to cook, and it makes enough chili for 4-6 servings.

Protein: 30.8g. Net Carbs: 7.1g. Fats: 32.5g. Calories: 449.
20 Smart Points.

Ingredients
- ✓ Chicken Thighs and Drumsticks (3lbs bone-in, skin-on)
- ✓ Poblano Peppers (1lb seeds and stems remove, and chopped)
- ✓ Tomatillos (.75lb quartered)
- ✓ Ground Cumin (1 T)
- ✓ Jalapenos (2 with stems removed, chopped)
- ✓ Anaheim Peppers (2 with stems and seeds removed, chopped)
- ✓ Garlic (6 cloves, peeled)
- ✓ White Onion (1 C or 250mL, chopped)
- ✓ Fresh Cilantro (.5C or 125mL)
- ✓ Corn Tortillas
- ✓ Worcestershire Sauce (1 T)

How to Make
1. Set the instant pot to the sauté setting and combine the chicken, peppers and spices.
2. Heat until everything is gently sizzling.
3. Seal the lid and then manually set the pot to high pressure before cooking for 15 minutes.
4. Perform a quick release method as per your manufacturer's instructions.
5. Remove the chicken and place it into a separate bowl.
6. Pour the remaining contents of your instant pot and all other ingredients you have left into a high-powered blender and blend everything until it comes together as a smooth, creamy gravy-style broth.
7. Remove any bones from the chicken, shred it, and then place it back into the sauce.
8. Serve topped with fresh cilantro.

Chorizo Chili

This recipe needs 5 minutes to prepare, 20 minutes to cook, and it will prepare enough chili for 10 servings.

Protein: 24g. Net Carbs: 12g. Fats: 22g. Calories: 335.
14 Smart Points.

Ingredients
- ✓ Bell Pepper (1 C or 250mL, chopped)
- ✓ Chorizo (2lbs)
- ✓ Onion (1 C or 250mL, chopped)
- ✓ Crushed Tomatoes (28oz can)
- ✓ Chilies (1.5 TSP, ground)
- ✓ Ground Cumin (1 TSP)
- ✓ Beef Broth (3 C or 750mL)
- ✓ Oil (1 T)
- ✓ Garlic Powder (1 TSP)
- ✓ Instant Coffee (.5 TSP)
- ✓ Cocoa Powder (.5 TSP)
- ✓ Black Soy Beans (15oz can, drained)

How to Make
1. Heat the oil in your instant pot using the sauté setting.
2. Brown the chorizo sausage before adding the onions and bell peppers.
3. Cook until soft, then add the spices to the pot.
4. Continue cooking for a few extra moments until the spices are aromatic.
5. Once you can smell the spices, add the broth, tomatoes, instant coffee, cocoa and black beans.
6. Manually set your instant pot to the high pressure setting and allow your chili to cook for 10 minutes.
7. Perform the quick release method recommended by your manufacturer.
8. Serve and enjoy.

Smoky Bacon Chili

This recipe needs 15 minutes to prepare, 50 minutes to cook, and will prepare a total of 4 servings of chili.

Protein: 28.2g. Net Carbs: 10.9g. Fats: 37.7g. Calories: 515.
23 Smart Points.

Ingredients

- ✓ Bacon (6 slices cut into 1-inch strips)
- ✓ Garlic (2 cloves, minced)
- ✓ Bell Pepper (2 C or 500mL, diced)
- ✓ Onion (1 C or 250mL, diced)
- ✓ Chili Powder (1 T)
- ✓ Ground Beef (1lb)
- ✓ Tomato Sauce (8oz can)
- ✓ Fire Roasted Tomatoes (14oz can)
- ✓ Garlic Powder (1 T)
- ✓ Cumin (2 TSP)
- ✓ Paprika (1 T)
- ✓ Cayenne Pepper (.5 TSP)

How to Make

1. Turn the instant pot to the sauté mode and sauté the bacon until it becomes crispy.
2. Leave the fat in the instant pot instead of using an alternative cooking oil for the remaining part of the cooking process.
3. In the remaining bacon fat, cook the onions, peppers and garlic.
4. Sauté these ingredients until the onions become translucent.
5. Add the remaining ingredients to the instant pot and mix thoroughly.
6. Cook for an additional 5 minutes on the sauté setting before adding the bacon back to the pot.
7. Secure the lid on your instant pot and turn it to medium pressure.
8. Cook your chili for 30 minutes and then let your instant pot do a natural release on its own.
9. When it's done, open the lid and mix your ingredients together well before serving.

Tomatillo Chili

This recipe needs 15 minutes to prepare, 35 minutes to cook, and it will prepare enough for 8 servings of chili.

Protein: 20g. Net Carbs: 6g. Fats: 23g. Calories: 325.
14 Smart Points.

Ingredients

- ✓ Ground Pork (1lb)
- ✓ Ground Beef (1lb)
- ✓ Chili Powder (1 T)
- ✓ Tomato Paste (6oz can)
- ✓ Garlic Powder (1 T)
- ✓ Onion (.5 C or 125mL, chopped)
- ✓ Tomatillos (.5 C or 125mL, chopped)
- ✓ Jalapeno (1 T, chopped)
- ✓ Ground Cumin (1 T)

How to Make

1. Use the sauté function on your instant pot to brown your ground meats.
2. Once browned, add the remaining ingredients to the instant pot and stir thoroughly so everything is combined.
3. Secure the lid on your instant pot and manually set it to the high-pressure setting.
4. Cook your chili for 35 minutes before allowing the pressure to naturally release.
5. When the release is done, serve your chili.

Asian Beef

Prep Time: 10 min. Cook Time: 45 min.
Yields: 12 Servings – 4 oz. each

Nutrition: 245 Cal., 38 g Prot., 9 g Fat, 0.0 g Net Carbs.
6 Smart Points.

Ingredients
- ✓ 1 (4-5 lb.) boneless chuck roast
- ✓ 3 crushed garlic cloves
- ✓ 1 t. of each:
  - o Crushed red pepper flakes
  - o Orange extract
- ✓ 2 tbsp. fresh ginger
- ✓ ¼ c. sugar-free fish sauce
- ✓ 2 tbsp. granulated sugar substitute – your favorite
- ✓ ½ c. water

Step # 1 (fixings)
- ✓ 1 tbsp. orange zest
- ✓ 1 t. red wine vinegar
- ✓ 1 tbsp. granulated sugar sweetener - favorite

Ingredients for the Toppings
- ✓ Butter lettuce leaves
- ✓ Shredded red cabbage
- ✓ Chopped Scallions
- ✓ Fresh orange zest
- ✓ Chopped cilantro

Ingredients for the Orange Sauce
- ✓ ½ t. fresh orange zest
- ✓ 1 t. Sriracha hot sauce
- ✓ ¼ c. sugar-free mayonnaise
- ✓ 1 t. granulated sugar alternative of choice

How to Make
1. Combine the roast with the rest of the fixings (in the first group) in your Instant Pot.
2. Secure the lid and set on the pot on high-pressure for 35 minutes.
3. Perform a natural release or quick release the pressure. Pour in the vinegar, sweetener and orange zest. Sauté for five minutes. Take it out of the pot.
4. Shred the chicken and add the options of your choice on the lettuce leaves or in a dish.
5. Prepare and serve with the sauce if desired.

Balsamic Beef Pot Roast

Prep Time: 10 min. Cooking Time: 55 min.
Yields: 10 Servings.

Nutrition: 393 Cal., 30 g Prot., 28 g Fat, 3 g Net Carbs.
10 Smart Points.

Ingredients
- ✓ 1 t. of each:
  - o Ground black pepper
  - o Garlic powder
- ✓ 1 tbsp. kosher salt
- ✓ 1 (3 lb.) boneless chuck roast
- ✓ ¼ c. balsamic vinegar
- ✓ ½ c. chopped onion
- ✓ 2 c. water
- ✓ ¼ t. xanthan gum
- ✓ For the Garnish: Chopped fresh parsley

How to Make
1. Slice the roast in half and season with the garlic powder, pepper and salt.
1. Prepare the pot using the sauté function and brown the meat.
2. Pour in the onion, water and vinegar. Secure the lid and set for 35 minutes.
3. Perform a natural release method to release the pressure in pot.
4. Add the meat to a container and break it apart.
5. Discard the fat and use the sauté function to simmer the juices in the pot.
6. Add the meat back after whisking in the xanthan gum.
7. Gently stir and turn off the heat.
8. Garnish as desired.

Barbacoa Beef

Prep Time: 15 min. Cook Time: 65 min.
Yields: 9 Servings – 4 oz. each.

Nutrition: 153 Cal., 24 g Prot., 4.5 g Fat, 2 g Net Carbs.
4 Smart Points.

Ingredients
- ✓ ½ med. onion
- ✓ 5 garlic cloves
- ✓ 2-4 chipotles in adobo sauce – to taste
- ✓ 1 lime – juiced
- ✓ 1 tbsp. ground of each:
  - ○ Cumin
  - ○ Oregano
- ✓ 1 c. water
- ✓ ½ t. ground cloves
- ✓ 3 bay leaves
- ✓ 2 ½ t. kosher salt
- ✓ Black pepper – to taste
- ✓ 3 lb. eye of round/bottom round – fat trimmed away
- ✓ 1 t. oil

How to Make
1. In a blender, puree the onion, garlic cloves, lime juice, water, cloves, chipotles, cumin and oregano – until smooth.
2. Remove all fat and chop into 3-inch bits. Season with 2 teaspoons of salt and a pinch of pepper.
3. Prepare the Instant Pot on the sauté setting and add the oil. Brown the meat into batches (5 min.).
4. Add the sauce from the blender along with the bay leaves into the Instant Pot.
5. Secure the lid and set the timer for 65 minutes using the high-pressure setting.
6. Perform a natural or quick release method to release the pressure.
7. Shred the beef with two forks. Reserve the juices and throw the bay leaves in the trash.
8. Return the meat to the pot with the cumin, salt to taste, and add 1 ½ cups of the reserved juices.
9. Serve when hot.

Beef Tips Stroganoff

Prep Time: 8 min. Cooking Time: 30 min.
Yields: 4 Servings.

Nutrition: 321 Cal., 33 g Prot., 16 g Fat, 7 g Net Carbs.
11 Smart Points.

Ingredients
- ✓ 1 tbsp. oil
- ✓ 1 tbsp. garlic
- ✓ ½ c. diced onions
- ✓ 1 lb. beef/pork stew meat
- ✓ 1 ½ c. chopped mushrooms
- ✓ 1 t. salt
- ✓ 1 tbsp. Worcestershire sauce
- ✓ ½ t. pepper to taste
- ✓ ¾ c. water

Ingredients to Finish
- ✓ ¼ t. arrowroot starch/cornstarch/xanthan gum
- ✓ 1/3 c. sour cream

How to Make
1. Prepare the Instant Pot using the sauté function.
2. Heat the oil and toss in the garlic and onions.
3. Stir for a one minute and add in all the ingredients except the sour cream.
4. Secure the lid and set on high pressure for 20 minutes.
5. Perform a natural release method.
6. Change the pot to the sauté function and stir in the sour cream.
7. Sprinkle in the xanthan gum slowly, stirring as it thickens.
8. Serve and enjoy with some low-carb noodles or cauliflower rice.

Braised Cubed Steak

Prep Time: 10 min. Cooking Time: 40 min.
Yields: 8 Servings.

Nutrition: 154 Cal., 23.5 g Prot., 5.5 g Fat, 3 g Net Carbs.
4 Smart Points.

Ingredients
- ✓ 1 c. water
- ✓ 8 cubed steaks – 28 oz. pkg.
- ✓ Black pepper to taste
- ✓ 1 ¾ t. garlic salt/adobo seasoning
- ✓ 1 can tomato sauce (8 oz.)
- ✓ 1/3 c. green pitted olives (+) 2 tbsp. of brine
- ✓ 1 small red pepper
- ✓ ½ med. onion

How to Make
1. Chop the peppers and onions into ¼-inch strips.
2. Prepare the beef with the salt/adobo and pepper.
3. Toss it into the Instant Pot along with the remainder of the ingredients.
4. Secure the top and prepare for 25 minutes under high pressure.
5. Perform a natural release method.
6. Serve and enjoy!

Cabbage & Corned Beef

Prep Time: 20 min. Cooking Time: 1 hr. 15 min.
Yields: 12 Servings.

Nutrition: 334 Cal., 23.7 g Prot., 22.8 g Fat, 5.5 g Net Carbs. **14 Smart Points.**

Ingredients
- ✓ 6 c. water
- ✓ 4 lb. corned beef brisket
- ✓ 4 garlic cloves
- ✓ 2 t. black peppercorns
- ✓ 2 t. dried mustard
- ✓ 1 c. sliced - 2 onions
- ✓ 1 c. chopped – 4 celery stalks
- ✓ 1 c. sliced – 4 carrots

How to Make
1. Discard the seasoning packet in the meat package.
2. Arrange the brisket in the Instant Pot.
3. Pour in the water (to cover the brisket) and add the spices.
4. Secure the lid and choose the meat/stew setting (high-60 min.).
5. Perform a natural release method (20 min.) and remove the brisket.
6. Place in the foil to keep it warm.
7. Stir in the veggies and choose the soup function on your pot (15 min.).
8. Perform a quick release and add the brisket to the pot. Enjoy!

Cheese & Steak Pot Roast

Prep Time: 25 min. Cook Time: 45-50 min.
Yields: Servings.

Nutrition: 425 Cal., 46.1 g Prot., 25.7 g Fat, 3.5 g Net Carbs. **16 Smart Points.**

Ingredients
- ✓ 1 tbsp. oil
- ✓ 2 large thinly sliced onions
- ✓ 8 oz. sliced mushrooms
- ✓ 1-2 tbsp. Montreal steak seasoning/another favorite Keto choice
- ✓ 1 tbsp. butter
- ✓ ½ c. beef stock
- ✓ 3 lb. chuck roast
- ✓ Optional: Keto cheese of choice – add the carbs

How to Make
1. Program your Instant Pot to the sauté mode and pour in the oil.
2. Rub the roast with the seasoning. Sauté for 1-2 minutes per side.
3. Remove and add the butter and onions.
4. Toss in the mushrooms, peppers, stock and roast.
5. Select the manual high-pressure setting for 35 minutes.
6. Perform a natural release method.
7. Shred the meat, sprinkle with cheese and serve as desired.

Chipotle Shredded Beef

Prep Time: 25 min. Cooking Time: 1 hr. 10 min.
Yields: 16 Servings or 4-5 Cups.

Nutrition: 334 Cal., 22.6 g Prot., 25.6 g Fat, 2.2 g Net Carbs. **15 Smart Points.**

Ingredients
- ✓ 1 t. black pepper
- ✓ 2 t. salt
- ✓ 3 lb. beef chuck roast
- ✓ 2 tbsp. olive oil
- ✓ 1 tbsp. adobo sauce – from chipotle with adobe can
- ✓ 1 chipotle in adobo – seeds removed or not – chopped
- ✓ 2 t. dried of each:
  - ○ Oregano
  - ○ Cumin
- ✓ ½ t. chili powder
- ✓ 1 c. fresh cilantro – roughly chopped
- ✓ 1 seeded green bell pepper – large chunks
- ✓ 1 peeled – quartered onion
- ✓ 1 c. water.

How to Make
1. Sprinkle the roast with the pepper and salt.
2. Select the Instant Pot sauté function and pour in the oil. Arrange the roast in the pot and sauté for 3-4 minutes on each side.
3. Spread the adobo sauce and chipotle pepper. Sprinkle the chili powder, oregano, and cumin. Toss the cilantro on top.
4. Add the peppers and onions. Pour the water into the pot.
5. Prepare for 60 minutes using the high-pressure setting.
6. Perform a natural release method and remove the meat. Shred with two forks and discard the veggies.
7. Add the beef back into the juices. Keep it warm until ready to serve.

Greek Meatballs with Tomato Sauce

Prep Time: 15 min. Cook Time: 25 min.
Yields: 6 Servings.

Nutrition: 261 Cal., 32g Prot., 20g Fat, g Net Carbs.
10 Smart Points.

Ingredients
- ✓ 1 slightly beaten egg
- ✓ 1 lb. ground beef
- ✓ ¼ c. chopped parsley
- ✓ ½ c. finely chopped onion
- ✓ 1/3 c. Arborio rice
- ✓ To Taste: Pepper and salt

Ingredients for the Sauce
- ✓ 1 c. water
- ✓ 14 oz. diced tomatoes
- ✓ ½ t. of each:
  - ○ -Smoked paprika
  - ○ -Cinnamon
- ✓ 1 t. dried oregano
- ✓ ¼ t. ground cloves
- ✓ To Taste: More pepper & salt

How to Make
1. Mix all the meatballs ingredients, shaping them into eight to ten balls.
2. Arrange them in a single layer inside the pot.
3. Mix the sauce components inside a dish and pour over the prepared meatballs.
4. Program the Instant Pot for 15 minutes using the high-pressure setting.
5. Release the pressure using the natural release method.
6. Remove the meatballs and blend the sauce until smooth using an immersion blender.
7. Pour over the meatballs, garnish, and serve.

Ground Beef with Coconut Milk & Spinach

Prep Time: 5 min. Cooking Time: 10 min.
Yields: 4 Servings.

Nutrition: 341 Cal., 21 g Prot., 23 g Fat, 7 g Net Carbs.
15 Smart Points.

Ingredients
- ✓ 1 lb. ground beef
- ✓ 2-inch knob of ginger – chopped
- ✓ 4 minced garlic cloves
- ✓ ½ onion – cut into halves and thinly sliced
- ✓ 1 t. garam masala
- ✓ 2 chopped tomatoes
- ✓ 2 bay leaves
- ✓ ½ t. cayenne pepper
- ✓ 1 t. of each:
  - ○ -Turmeric
  - ○ -Salt
- ✓ Cinnamon stick
- ✓ 2-3 green cardamom pods
- ✓ ½ c. water

Optional
- ✓ 1 t. ground ginger
- ✓ 1 tbsp. ground fennel seeds
- ✓ 1 t. Indian black salt
- ✓ 1 c. peas

How to Make
1. Select the Instant Pot sauté function and brown the beef.
2. Add all the ingredients (except for the peas).
3. Program the pot to high pressure for 10 minutes.
4. Perform a natural release method for 10 minutes when the time has elapsed.
5. Add the peas, stir and enjoy!

Indian Keema

Prep Time: 20 min. Cook Time: 10 min.
Yields: 4 Servings.

Nutrition: 334 Cal., 29 g Prot., 20 g Fat, 4 g Net Carbs.
13 Smart Points.

Ingredients
- ✓ 1 c. chopped onion
- ✓ 1 tbsp. ghee/oil
- ✓ 1 tbsp. of each:
  - ○ -Garlic
  - ○ -Minced ginger
- ✓ 4 pods white/green cardamom
- ✓ 3-4 pieces cinnamon sticks
- ✓ 1 lb. ground beef
- ✓ ½ t. of each:
  - ○ -Cumin
  - ○ -Ground coriander
  - ○ -Turmeric
  - ○ -Cayenne pepper
- ✓ 1 t. of each:
  - ○ -Salt
  - ○ -Garam masala
- ✓ ¼ c. water

How to Make
1. Pour the oil into the Instant Pot. When it's hot, add the ghee/oil.
2. Toss in the cardamom and cinnamon.
3. Sauté for 10 seconds.
4. Toss in the garlic, ginger, and onions, sautéing for three to five minutes.
5. Blend in the beef and sauté for three to four minutes.
6. Add the water and spices.
7. Secure the lid and cook on high for five minutes.
8. Perform a natural release for 10 minutes.
9. Perform a quick release after that to release the remaining steam.
10. Serve and enjoy!

Italian Meatballs

Prep Time: 10 min. Cooking Time: 25 min.
Yields: 5 Servings.

Nutrition: 455 Cal., 34 g Prot., 33 g Fat, 5 g Net Carbs.
19 Smart Points.

Ingredients for the Meatballs
- ✓ 1 ½ lb. ground beef – lean
- ✓ 2 tbsp. freshly chopped parsley
- ✓ 2 eggs
- ✓ ½ c. almond flour
- ✓ ¾ c. grated parmesan cheese
- ✓ ¼ t. of each:
  - ○ -Garlic Powder
  - ○ -Ground black pepper
- ✓ 1 t. of each:
  - ○ -Kosher salt
  - ○ -Dried onion flakes
- ✓ 1/3 c. warm water
- ✓ ¼ t. dried oregano

Cooking Ingredients
- ✓ 1 t. olive oil
- ✓ 3 c. 'keto' marinara sauce/sugar-free sauce

How to Make
1. Mix all the meatball ingredients and shape them into 15 (2-inch) balls.
2. Add the oil to the Instant Pot and select the sauté function.
3. Brown the meatballs by leaving a ½-inch space between each one inside the pot. You can also brown them in a skillet first.
4. Pour in the marinara sauce and secure the lid.
5. Cook on low-pressure for 10 minutes.
6. Perform a natural release method to release the pressure.
7. Serve and enjoy.

Picadillo in the Pot

Prep Time: 5 min. Cooking Time: 25 min.
Yields: 6 Servings.

Nutrition: 207 Cal., 25 g Prot., 8.5 g Fat, 4 g Net Carbs.
7 Smart Points.

Ingredients

- ✓ 1 ½ lb. lean ground beef
- ✓ 2 minced garlic cloves
- ✓ ½ large chopped onion
- ✓ 1 t. kosher salt
- ✓ 1 chopped tomato
- ✓ ½ finely chopped red bell pepper
- ✓ 2 tbsp. cilantro
- ✓ ½ of a can (4 oz.) tomato sauce – ex. Goya
- ✓ 1 t. ground cumin
- ✓ 1-2 bay leaves
- ✓ 2 tbsp. green olives/capers/alcaparrado
- ✓ 2 tbsp. of brine (juice from olives)
- ✓ 3 tbsp. water

How to Make

1. Select the sauté function on your Instant Pot and place the meat, salt and pepper in the bottom to brown.
2. Toss in the garlic onion, tomato and cilantro.
3. Sauté for one minute and add the olives, brine, bay leaf and cumin.
4. Pour in the sauce with the water and stir.
5. Secure the lid for 15 minutes under high pressure.
6. Perform a natural or quick release method.
7. Serve and enjoy.

Shepherd's Pie

Prep Time: 25 min. Cooking Time: 20 min.
Yields: 12 Servings.

Nutrition: 303 Cal., 21.5 g Prot., 21.2 g Fat,
4.1 g Net Carbs. **13 Smart Points.**

Ingredients

- ✓ 1 c. water
- ✓ 4 tbsp. butter
- ✓ 1 head cauliflower
- ✓ 4 oz. cream cheese
- ✓ 1 c. mozzarella
- ✓ 1 egg
- ✓ Pepper & Salt to taste
- ✓ 1 tbsp. garlic powder
- ✓ 2 lb. ground beef
- ✓ 2 c. of each:
    - ○ Frozen peas
    - ○ Frozen carrots
- ✓ 8 oz. sliced mushrooms
- ✓ 1 c. beef broth

How to Make

1. Pour the water into the Instant Pot and arrange the cauliflower on top with the leaves and stems removed.
2. Close the lid and set for 5 minutes using the high-pressure mode.
3. Perform a quick release method and add the cauliflower to a blender.
4. Add the cream cheese, butter, mozzarella, egg, pepper and salt. Blend until smooth.
5. Drain the water from the Instant Pot.
6. Toss in the beef, carrots, peas, garlic powder, and broth with a bit more pepper and salt to your liking.
7. Blend in the cauliflower mixture and cook for 10 minutes on high (manual function).
8. Serve and enjoy!

Beef Ribs

This recipe needs 15 minutes to prepare, 35 minutes to cook, and will prepare enough for 1 serving.

Protein: 8.7g. Net Carbs: 5g. Fats: 21g. Calories: 184.
10 Smart Points.

Ingredients

- ✓ 3 cloves garlic
- ✓ 1 onion quartered
- ✓ 1 tbsp olive oil
- ✓ 4 lbs/1800g beef short ribs

How to Make

1. Sprinkle the ribs with salt.
2. Set your instant pot to sauté mode.
3. Add the oil and heat until its warm.
4. Brown the ribs after the oil has been heated.
5. Once the ribs have been browned, place them into the instant pot.
6. Add the water, garlic and onions.
7. Close and seal the lid.
8. Set the instant pot on manual and cook for 35 minutes.
9. When finished, perform a quick release on your instant pot to release the pressure inside.
10. Serve & Enjoy!

Balsamic Beef Roast

This recipe needs 15 minutes to prepare, 90 minutes to cook and will prepare enough for 1 serving.

Protein: 30g. Net Carbs: 3g. Fats: 28g. Calories: 393.
17 Smart Points.

Ingredients

- ✓ ¼ tsp xanthan gum
- ✓ ½ cup/113g chopped onion
- ✓ 2 cups/450g water
- ✓ ¼ cup/57g balsamic vinegar
- ✓ 1 tsp garlic powder
- ✓ 1 tsp black pepper
- ✓ 1 tbsp salt
- ✓ 3 lb/1370g boneless chuck roast

How to Make

1. Cut the beef roast in half.
2. Season it with garlic powder, pepper and salt.
3. Set your instant pot to sauté mode.
4. Brown the roast on all sides.
5. Add ½ cup onion, 1 cup water and ¼ cup balsamic vinegar to the beef.
6. Cover it and seal the lid on your instant pot. Set it on manual for 35 minutes.
7. When finished, release the pressure naturally.
8. Open the lid and remove the beef.
9. Shred it with two forks and discard the fat.
10. Turn your instant pot to sauté mode and bring the liquid at the bottom to the boil. Simmer for ten minutes.
11. Whisk in the xanthan gum.
12. Add the beef back in and gently stir.
13. Turn off the heat and serve as you would like.

Moroccan Beef

This recipe needs 15 minutes to prepare, 10 hours to cook and it will prepare enough for 1 serving.

Protein: 4g. Net Carbs: 4g. Fats: 20g. Calories: 218.
12 Smart Points.

Ingredients

- ✓ 1 tsp salt
- ✓ 4 tbsp garam masala
- ✓ 2 lbs/900g beef roasts
- ✓ ½ cup/125ml sliced onion

How to Make

1. Slice the onions into strips.
2. Put them into the bottom of your instant pot.
3. Place the roast on top of the onions.
4. Add in the salt and spices.
5. Cover. Set on low and cook for 8 hours.
6. Remove the roast and shred it with forks.
7. Cook for another 2 hours to let the spices marinate into the meat.
8. Serve with tortillas & enjoy!

Asian Pot Roast

This recipe needs 5 minutes to prepare, 45 minutes to cook and will make enough pot roast for 12 servings.

Protein: 38g. Net Carbs: 0g. Fat: 9g. Calories: 245.
6 Smart Points.

Ingredients

- ✓ Boneless Chuck Roast (4-5lb size)
- ✓ Ginger (2 T, grated)
- ✓ Garlic (3 cloves, crushed)
- ✓ Orange Extract (1 TSP)
- ✓ Sugar-Free Fish Sauce (.25 C or 65mL)
- ✓ Granulated Sugar Substitute (such as Swerve) (3 T, divided)
- ✓ Water (.5 cup or 125mL)
- ✓ Red Wine Vinegar (1 TSP)
- ✓ Red Pepper Flakes (1 TSP, crushed)
- ✓ Orange Zest (1 T)

How to Make

1. Combine the chuck roast, fish sauce, orange extract, garlic, 2 T of sweetener, ginger, water and red pepper flakes in your instant pot.
2. Manually set your instant pot to high pressure for 35 minutes and cook.
3. When done, use the quick pressure release method as outlined in your manufacturer's guide.
4. Add the remaining sweetener, orange zest and red wine vinegar to the instant pot and stir.
5. Switch your instant pot to the sauté mode and cook for an additional 5 minutes.
6. Serve & enjoy!

Beef Stroganoff

This recipe needs 5 minutes to prepare, 30 minutes to cook and it will prepare enough beef stroganoff for 4 servings.

Protein: 33g. Net Carbs: 9g. Fats: 16g. Calories: 321.
11 Smart Points.

Ingredients
- ✓ Onions (.5 C or 125mL, diced)
- ✓ Garlic (1 T)
- ✓ Beef Stew Meat (1lb)
- ✓ Oil (1 T)
- ✓ Water (.75 C or 190mL)
- ✓ Mushrooms (1.5 C or 375mL, chopped)
- ✓ Worcestershire Sauce (1 T)
- ✓ Sour Cream (.33 C or 85mL)
- ✓ Corn Starch (.25 TSP)

How to Make
1. Begin by turning your instant pot to the sauté mode and melt the oil.
2. Sauté your garlic and onions until they become translucent.
3. Except for the corn starch and sour cream, pour all the remaining ingredients into your instant pot.
4. Manually set the pot to high pressure and cook for 20 minutes.
5. Perform a natural release method.
6. Open the lid and stir in the remaining ingredients.
7. Turn the instant pot to sauté mode and continue stirring until everything is mixed and creamy.
8. Serve over cauliflower rice.

Corned Beef & Cabbage

This recipe needs 15 minutes to prepare, 1 hour 15 minutes to cook and will prepare enough corned beef and cabbage to serve 12.

Protein: 23.7g. Net Carbs: 8.1g. Fats: 22.8g. Calories: 334.
14 Smart Points.

Ingredients
- ✓ Corned Beef Brisket (4-5lb)
- ✓ Black Peppercorns (2 TSP)
- ✓ Dried Mustard (2 TSP)
- ✓ Cabbage (8 C or 2,000mL)
- ✓ Water (6 C or 1,500mL)
- ✓ Garlic (4 cloves)
- ✓ Onion (1 C or 250mL, sliced)
- ✓ Celery Stalks (1 C or 250mL, chopped)
- ✓ Carrots (1 C or 250mL, cubed)

How to Make
1. Place the corned beef and water in your instant pot.
2. Turn the instant pot to "Meat/Stew" setting, or manually set it to high pressure.
3. Cook the beef for 60 minutes.
4. Allow the instant pot to naturally release before removing the lid and brisket.
5. Add the vegetables.
6. Keep the brisket warm while you cook the vegetables for 15 minutes on the Sauté setting on your instant pot.
7. Perform a quick release method as per your manufacturer's instructions.
8. Add the beef back into the pot and choose the Sauté setting to ensure that all ingredients are at the same temperature before serving.
9. Enjoy!

No Noodle Lasagne

This recipe needs 10 minutes to prepare, 25 minutes to cook, and will make enough lasagna for 8 servings.

Protein: 36g. Net Carbs: 7.9g. Fats: 3.2g. Calories: 339.
8 Smart Points.

Ingredients
- ✓ Garlic (2 cloves, minced)
- ✓ Onion (.5 C or 125mL, sliced)
- ✓ Ground Beef (1lb)
- ✓ Parmesan Cheese (.5 C or 125mL)
- ✓ Ricotta Cheese (1.5 C or 375mL)
- ✓ Marinara Sauce (25oz jar)
- ✓ Mozzarella (8oz, sliced)
- ✓ Egg (1 large)

How to Make
1. Begin by browning the beef and garlic in your instant pot using the sauté mode.
2. In the meantime, combine the parmesan, egg and cheese in a bowl until thoroughly blended.
3. Blend in the marinara sauce and browned beef, and then remove half of it.
4. Spread a generous layer of about half of the mozzarella, then top that with the ricotta cheese mixture.
5. Add this back to the remaining marinara meat sauce, then top again with mozzarella and ricotta cheese.
6. To avoid condensation drips, put a layer of tinfoil over the lasagna before manually setting it to high pressure and cooking it for 8-10 minutes in your instant pot. This will help ensure that the cheese crisps. If you do not mind a runnier cheese, do not worry about this part.
7. Perform a quick release method, sprinkle additional dusting of parmesan cheese over the lasagna and let it sit for about 10 minutes before serving.
8. Enjoy!

Belizean Stewed Chicken

Prep Time & Cooking Time Vary Depending on time marinated. Yields: 8 Servings – 1 piece of chicken and ¼ c. of the sauce.

Nutrition: 319 Cal., 28 g Prot., 22 g Fat, 3 g Net Carbs.
13 Smart Points.

Ingredients
- ✓ 1 tbsp. coconut oil
- ✓ 4 whole chicken legs – thighs and drumsticks
- ✓ 3 tbsp. organic or homemade Worcestershire sauce
- ✓ 2 tbsp. of each:
  - o -Recado rojo or achiote seasoning/paste
  - o -White vinegar
- ✓ 1 c. sliced yellow onions
- ✓ 3 sliced garlic cloves
- ✓ 1 t. of each:
  - o -Dried oregano - Mexican
  - o -Ground cumin
- ✓ 1 tbsp. granulated sugar substitute – ex. erythritol
- ✓ ½ t. ground black pepper
- ✓ 2 c. chicken stock

How to Make
1. Combine the recado rojo or achiote seasoning/paste, cumin, oregano, Worcestershire sauce, vinegar and pepper.
2. Stir well and add the pieces of chicken, rubbing it into the skin.
3. Marinate for a minimum of one hour or overnight. Reserve the marinade.
4. Set your Instant Pot to sauté mode and add the oil.
5. Prepare the chicken in batches for two minutes per side. Place it on a platter.
6. Sauté the onions and garlic for two to three minutes in the Instant Pot. Toss in the chicken.
7. Add the broth/marinade over the chicken and seal the pot.
8. Set the timer for 20 minutes under high pressure.
9. Perform a quick release method.
10. Serve and garnish as desired.

Sesame Chicken

Prep Time: 5 min. Cooking Time: 25 min.
Yields: 8 Servings.

Nutrition: 443 Calories, 20 g Protein, 37 g Fat, 1 g Net Carbs. **22 Smart Points.**

Ingredients

- ✓ ½ c. sesame oil
- ✓ 2.2 lb. chicken wings/thighs
- ✓ 1 oz. julienned ginger
- ✓ 2 tbsp. oil – to sauté
- ✓ 6-8 tbsp. Shaoxing Wine to taste
- ✓ 2 ½ t. light soy sauce
- ✓ ¾ c. water
- ✓ 2 t. dark soy sauce

How to Make

1. Prepare the chicken with a mixture of the two soy sauces.
2. Select the sauté mode and add the oil.
3. Sauté the ginger and deglaze the Instant Pot with the water.
4. Arrange the chicken in the pot with the rest of the oil and water. Secure the lid.
5. Cook for six minutes using the high-pressure function.
6. Perform a natural release method for 10 minutes and a quick release method after that to release the remaining steam.
7. Transfer the chicken to a platter.
8. Using the sauté function, add the wine and cook slowly for two to three minutes.
9. Garnish with some cilantro and enjoy hot.

Taiwanese Chicken

Preparation Time: 5 min. Cooking Time: 10 min.
Yields: 6 Servings.

Nutrition: 307 Calories, 31 g Protein, 15 g Fat, 7 g Net Carbs. **10 Smart Points.**

Ingredients

- ✓ 6 dried red chilis
- ✓ ¼ c. sesame oil
- ✓ 2 tbsp. ginger
- ✓ *To Taste: Salt*
- ✓ ¼ c. of each:
  - o Minced garlic
  - o Rice wine/Pale dry sherry
  - o Soy sauce

For the Finish

- ✓ ½ t. xanthan gum
- ✓ ¼ c. Thai basil - chopped

How to Make

1. Prepare the Instant Pot using the sauté setting.
2. Toss in the ginger, chilis and garlic.
3. Sauté for two minutes and add the rest of the fixings.
4. Cook for seven minutes and perform a natural release method for ten minutes. Open the lid and add the basil.
5. Stir until it boils. Sprinkle in the xanthan gum.
6. Add the cornstarch if a thickener consistency is needed.
7. Serve and enjoy!

Bruschetta Chicken

Prep Time: 15 min. Cook Time: 44 min.
Yields: 4 Servings – 8 oz. each.

Nutrition: 480 Cal., 52 g Prot., 26 g Fat, 4 g Net Carbs.
18 Smart Points.

Ingredients
- ✓ 2 tbsp. balsamic vinegar
- ✓ 2 t. minced garlic cloves
- ✓ 1 t. black pepper
- ✓ ½ t. sea salt
- ✓ 1/3 c. olive oil
- ✓ ½ c. sun-dried tomatoes in olive oil
- ✓ 2 lb. chicken breasts – quartered – boneless
- ✓ 2 tbsp. chopped fresh basil

How to Make
1. Whisk the vinegar, oil, garlic, pepper and salt together.
2. Fold in the tomatoes and basil.
3. Put the breasts in a freezer bag with the mixture for 30 minutes.
4. Add all the ingredients into your Instant Pot and secure the lid.
5. Select the poultry setting (9 min.).
6. Perform a natural release method to release the pressure for five minutes, and a quick release after that to release the remaining steam
7. Serve and enjoy!

Creamy Chicken

Time: 10 min. Cook Time: 20 min.
Yields: 4 Servings.

Nutrition: 405 Cal., 21 g Prot., 31 g Fat, 9 g Net Carbs.
19 Smart Points.

Ingredients for the Sauce
- ✓ 6 garlic cloves
- ✓ 1 chopped onion
- ✓ 1 to 2-inch knots of ginger
- ✓ ½ c. full-fat coconut milk
- ✓ 1 tbsp. powdered chicken broth base
- ✓ 1 can (10 oz.) Rotel canned tomato and chilis
- ✓ 1 t. ground turmeric

Ingredients for the Chicken
- ✓ 1 ½ c. chopped celery
- ✓ 2 c. chopped Swiss chard
- ✓ 1 lb. chicken thighs

Ingredient for the Finish:
- ✓ ½ c. full-fat coconut milk

How to Make
1. Pour the coconut milk, broth base, turmeric, garlic, onion, ginger, tomatoes, and chilis into a blender.
2. Roughly puree into chunks and add them into the Instant Pot.
3. Toss them in the celery, chard and chopped chicken.
4. Select the Sauté setting on your pot (5 min. high pressure).
5. Perform a natural release method for ten minutes, and quick release the rest.
6. Pour in the remainder of the coconut milk, stir, and enjoy.

Creamy Salsa Chicken

Time: 10 min. Cook Time: 20 min.
Yields: 6 Servings.

Nutrition: 529 Cal., 70.7 g Prot., 23.9 g Fat, 3.3 g Net Carbs. **16 Smart Points.**

Ingredients
- ✓ ½ c. chicken broth
- ✓ 2 ½ - 3 lb. chicken breasts
- ✓ 4 oz. cream cheese
- ✓ 1 c. salsa
- ✓ ½ c. cottage cheese
- ✓ 1-2 t. fajita/taco seasoning

Optional Garnishes
- ✓ Sour cream
- ✓ Shredded cheese
- ✓ Chopped tomatoes
- ✓ Avocado
- ✓ Cilantro

How to Make
1. Arrange the chicken in the Instant Pot with the broth.
2. Prepare on the poultry setting (10 min.).
3. Perform a quick release, making sure the chicken is a minimum temperature of 160ºF.
4. When done, place in a large container and reserve ½ cup of the juices.
5. Add the rest of the ingredients and ½ cup of broth to the pot.
6. Select the sauté function and whisk the cottage cheese and cream cheese well – until melted.
7. Shred the chicken and add it to the sauce
8. Serve and garnish to your liking.

French Garlic Chicken

Time: 10 min. Cook Time: 20 min.
Yields: 4 Servings.

Nutrition: 429 Cal., 19 g Prot., 37 g Fat, 4 g Net Carbs. **19 Smart Points.**

Ingredients for the Marinade
- ✓ 2 t. Herbes de Provence
- ✓ 2 tbsp. olive oil
- ✓ 1 tbsp. of each:
  - o Cider vinegar
  - o Prepared Dijon mustard
  - o Minced garlic
- ✓ 1 t. of each:
  - o Pepper
  - o Salt
- ✓ 1 lb. chicken thighs – no bones or skin

Other Ingredients
- ✓ 8 chopped garlic cloves
- ✓ 2 tbsp. butter
- ✓ ¼ c. of each:
  - o Cream
  - o Water

How to Make
1. Prepare the Marinade: Add all the ingredients using a whisk.
2. Add the chicken and marinate for 30 minutes at room temperature or in a fridge.
3. Select the sauté button on your pot and add the butter to melt.
4. Sauté the garlic for 2-3 minutes.
5. Toss in the chicken. Reserve the marinade. Lightly brown the chicken.
6. Pour in the water and marinade into the pot and secure the lid.
7. Cook for 10 minutes and check the temperature. Internal temperature must be 165ºF.
8. Transfer the chicken to a plate and add the cream to the Instant Pot, mixing well.
9. Pour the sauce over the chicken and enjoy.

Frozen Chicken Breasts

Prep Time: 2 min. Cooking Time: 35 min.
Yields: 4 Servings.

Nutrition: 128 Cal., 23 g Prot., 2 g Fat, 0 g Net Carbs.
2 Smart Points.

Ingredients
- ✓ 1 ¼ c. water
- ✓ 4 chicken breasts – skinless

How to Make
1. Pour the water into your Instant Pot and add the frozen chicken.
2. Secure the top and set for 10 minutes.
3. Perform a natural release for ten minutes, and a quick release after that to release the remaining steam.
4. Open the lid and enjoy!

Lemon Rotisserie Chicken

Time: 5 min. Cook Time: 34 min.
Yields: 6 Servings.

Nutrition: 284 Cal., 25.7 g Prot., 18.8 g Fat, 2.9 g Net Carbs. **11 Smart Points.**

Ingredients
- ✓ 2 tbsp. olive oil
- ✓ 4 lemon wedges – 1 lemon
- ✓ 1 ½ t. salt
- ✓ 1 t. of each:
- ✓ -Paprika
- ✓ -Garlic powder
- ✓ ½ t. ground black pepper
- ✓ 2.5 lb. whole chicken
- ✓ 1 c. chicken broth

How to Make
1. Wash the chicken and dry it with a paper towel. Insert the lemon wedges into the cavity of the bird.
2. Choose the sauté function on your Instant Pot.
3. Combine the pepper, garlic powder, salt, oil and paprika inside a dish.
4. Rub the top of the chicken (breast side down) using ½ of the spice mixture.
5. Sauté for three to four minutes.
6. Rub the rest on the other half and flip, cooking for up to one more minute.
7. Transfer the chicken to a container and add the trivet to the pot.
8. Put the chicken back (breast side down) and cover with the broth.
9. Secure the lid and set the timer for 20 minutes.
10. Perform a natural release method.
11. Serve and enjoy!

Salsa Shredded Chicken

Prep Time: 5 min. Cook Time: 30 min.
Yields: 5 Servings.

Nutrition: 125 Cal., 22 g Prot., 3 g Fat, 2 g Net Carbs.
2 Smart Points.

Ingredients
- ✓ 1 lb. chicken breast – skin & bones removed
- ✓ ¾ t. cumin
- ✓ ½ t. kosher salt
- ✓ Pinch of oregano
- ✓ Black pepper to taste
- ✓ 1 c. chunky salsa – homemade or favorite Keto version

How to Make
1. Sprinkle the chicken with the spices and add it to your Instant Pot.
2. Cover with the salsa and close the lid.
3. Cook for 20 minutes
4. Perform a natural or quick release method.
5. Add the chicken to a platter and shred.
6. Serve and enjoy!

Sesame Ginger Chicken

Prep Time: 5 min. Cook Time: 25 min.
Yields: 6 Servings.

Nutrition: 286 Cal., 21g Prot., 21 g Fat, 3 g Net Carbs
12 Smart Points.

Ingredients
- ✓ 1 ½ lb. chicken thighs – no skin or bones
- ✓ 2 tbsp. liquid aminos
- ✓ 1 tbsp. of each:
  - ○ Agave/another sweetener
  - ○ Minced ginger
  - ○ Minced garlic
  - ○ Sesame oil
  - ○ Rice vinegar

Salad Ingredients
- ✓ Julienned Carrots
- ✓ Julienned Cucumbers
- ✓ Red sliced onions - in rings

How to Make
1. Slice the chicken thighs into large chunks and combine them with the rest of the ingredients inside a heat-safe dish. Place foil over the dish.
2. Add two cups of water to the cooker. Place the steamer rack and bowl on top.
3. Program your Instant Pot for 10 minutes on high pressure/
4. Perform a 10-minute natural release and then perform a quick release to release the remaining pressure.
5. Shred the chicken and enjoy with the salad.

Thai Green Chicken Curry

Prep Time: 15 min. Cooking Time:8 hrs.
Yields: 6 Servings.

Nutrition: 231 Cal. ,17 g Prot., 15 g Fat, 5 g Net Carbs. **9 Smart Points.**

Ingredients

- ✓ 1 lb. chicken thighs – remove skin & bones
- ✓ 2 tbsp. curry paste
- ✓ 1 tbsp. of each:
  - o Coconut oil
  - o Minced garlic
  - o Minced ginger
- ✓ ½ c. sliced onion
- ✓ 2 c. peeled – chopped eggplant
- ✓ ½ c. basil leaves
- ✓ 1 chopped yellow, green or orange pepper
- ✓ 1 c. unsweetened coconut milk
- ✓ 2 tbsp. of each:
  - o Splenda/another sweetener
  - o Soy sauce/coconut aminos
- ✓ 1 tbsp. of each:
  - o Salt
  - o Fish sauce

How to Make

1. Set your Instant Pot on the sauté function. When hot, add the oil and curry paste. Sauté for one to two minutes.
2. Toss in the garlic and ginger – sear for about 30 seconds.
3. Stir in the onions along with the rest of the ingredients. Deglaze the pan.
4. Select the slow cooker mode on your instant pot and cook for 8 hours using a medium setting.
5. Stir and enjoy!

Whole Chicken & Gravy

Prep Time: 5 min. Cook Time: 40 min.
Yields: 12 Servings.

Nutrition:450 Cal., 34.5 g Prot., 30.2 g Fat, 0.7 g Net Carbs. **18 Smart Points.**

Ingredients

- ✓ 6 ½ lb. whole chicken
- ✓ 2 tbsp. olive oil
- ✓ ½ t. of each:
  - o Garlic powder
  - o Onion powder
  - o Black pepper
  - o Salt
- ✓ 1 t. dried Italian seasonings
- ✓ 1 ½ c. chicken broth (low-sodium)
- ✓ 2 t. guar gum

How to Make

1. Rub one tbsp. of oil over the chicken and add the rest of the oil into the Instant Pot.
2. Combine the dry seasonings and sprinkle them over the chicken.
3. Use the sauté function to warm the oil and add the chicken breast side down. Let it sauté for five minutes
4. Flip and put the chicken into the chicken broth.
5. Secure the top and set the timer for 40 minutes (manually).
6. When done, perform a quick release method.
7. Add the chicken to a bowl and prepare the gravy with the guar gum in the hot broth.
8. Stir until thickened. You can add another teaspoon if it isn't as thick as you would like.
9. Serve with gravy and a sprinkle of chopped parsley.

'Bo Ssäm' Style Pork & Noodle

Prep Time: 10 min. Cook Time: 10 min.
Yields: 6 Servings.

Nutrition: 296 Cal., 22 g Prot., 20 g Fat, 8 g Net Carbs.
12 Smart Points.

Ingredients for the Sauce
- ✓ 2 tbsp. gochujang paste
- ✓ 1 tbsp. of each:
  - ○ Soy sauce/organic coconut aminos
  - ○ Garlic powder
  - ○ Minced garlic
  - ○ Bean paste/doubanjiang
- ✓ 1 t. hot sesame oil – optional
- ✓ ½ t. ground Sichuan peppercorns
- ✓ 1 t. salt
- ✓ ¼ c. water

Other Ingredients
- ✓ 1 lb. ground pork
- ✓ 4-6 c./1 bunch bok choy

How to Make
1. Prepare your Instant Pot using the sauté function and add one tablespoon of oil. Toss in the pork and cook .
2. Combine the sauce ingredients.
3. Add the water and sauce to deglaze the pan.
4. Toss in the bok choy and set your pot to a high pressure setting for four minutes.
5. Perform a quick release method and serve with the prepared sauce.

Smothered Pork Chops

Prep Time: 10 min. Cooking Time: 42 min.
Yields: 4 Servings.

Nutrition: 481 Calories, 15g Protein, 33g Fat, 14g, Net Carbs 6g. **22 Smart Points.**

Ingredients
- ✓ 4 (4-6 oz.) pork loin chops – no bones
- ✓ 1 tbsp. paprika
- ✓ 1 t. of each:
  - ○ Black pepper
  - ○ Salt
  - ○ Onion powder
  - ○ Garlic powder
- ✓ ¼ t. cayenne pepper
- ✓ ½ med. sliced onion
- ✓ 6 oz. baby mushrooms – sliced
- ✓ 1 tbsp. butter
- ✓ ¼ t. xanthan gum
- ✓ ½ c. heavy cream
- ✓ 1 tbsp. chopped fresh parsley
- ✓ 2 tbsp. coconut oil

How to Make
1. Combine the onion powder, paprika, garlic powder, cayenne, salt and pepper together.
2. Rinse and dry the pork. Sprinkle with one tablespoon of the mixture, saving the rest for later.
3. Warm the oil in the Instant Pot using the sauté function.
4. Add the chops to sauté for 3 minutes each side.
5. Remove the chops and add the onions and mushrooms. Top this off with the chops to cook slowly for 25 minutes longer
6. Perform a natural or quick release method.
7. Sprinkle ¼ of the xanthan gum into the juices and whisk. Add the butter. Once it's melted, add the sauce and simmer until it thickens.
8. Turn off the pot and add the rest of the xanthan gum until the desired consistency is met.
9. Serve the chops with a layer of gravy.

Chipotle Pork Roast

Prep Time: 21 min. Cook Time: 1 hr.
Yields: 4 Servings.

Nutrition: 460 Cal., 40 g Prot., 31.0 g Fat, 4 g Net Carbs.
19 Smart Points.

Ingredients
- ✓ 7 ¼ oz. diced tomatoes - canned
- ✓ 6 oz. bone broth
- ✓ 2 oz. mild diced canned green chilis
- ✓ 2 lb. pork roast
- ✓ ½ t. of each:
  - o -Cumin
  - o Onion powder
- ✓ 1 t. chipotle powder

How to Make
1. Combine all the ingredients in your Instant Pot.
2. Close the top of the pot and use the manual setting for 60 minutes.
3. Perform a natural release method.
4. Serve and enjoy.

Korean Spicy Pork

Prep Time: 10 min. Cook Time: 30 min.
Yields: 4 Servings.

Nutrition: 189 Cal., 15 g Prot., 9 g Fat, 9 g Net Carbs.
7 Smart Points.

Ingredients
- ✓ 1 lb. pork shoulder
- ✓ 1 thinly sliced onion
- ✓ 1 tbsp. of each:
  - - Minced garlic
  - - Minced ginger
  - - Soy sauce
  - - Sesame oil
  - - Rice wine
- ✓ 2 Splenda packs
- ✓ 1 t. Cayenne
- ✓ 2 tbsp. gochugaru
- ✓ ¼ c. water

Ingredients for Finishing
- ✓ ¼ c. sliced green onion
- ✓ 1 tbsp. sesame seeds
- ✓ 1 thinly sliced onion

How to Make
1. Cut the pork into ¼ - ½- inch slices and add the rest of the marinade ingredients into a container.
2. Let this rest for 1 hour to 24 hours.
3. When ready to cook, use the high-pressure setting for 20 minutes.
4. Perform a natural release method.
5. Use a cast iron skillet to cook the thinly sliced onion and pork cubes.
6. Once the pan is hot, just empty in the sauce and mix with the pork.
7. When the sauce has cooled, the onions should be soft.
8. Toss in the green onions and sesame seeds and serve.

Mexican Pork Carnitas

Prep Time: 10 min. Cook Time: 65 min. approx.
Yields: 11 Servings.

Nutrition: 160 Cal., 20 g Prot., 7 g Fat, 1 g Net Carbs.
5 Smart Points.

Ingredients

- ✓ 2 ½ lb. shoulder blade roast – trimmed and boneless
- ✓ 2 t. kosher salt
- ✓ Black pepper – to your liking
- ✓ 1 ½ t. cumin
- ✓ 6 minced garlic cloves
- ✓ ½ t. sazon GOYA
- ✓ ¼ t. dry oregano
- ✓ ¾ c. reduced-sodium chicken broth/homemade
- ✓ 2 bay leaves
- ✓ 2-3 chipotle peppers in adobo sauce – to taste
- ✓ ¼ t. dry adobo seasoning – ex. Goya
- ✓ ½ t. garlic powder

How to Make

1. Prepare the roast with pepper and salt. Sear it for about 5 minutes in a skillet.
2. Let it cool and insert the garlic slivers into the roast using a blade (approximately one-inch deep).
3. Season with the garlic powder, sazon, cumin, oregano and adobo.
4. Arrange the chicken in the Instant Pot and add the broth, chipotle peppers and bay leaves.
5. Stir and secure the lid. Prepare using a high-pressure mode for 50 minutes (meat button).
6. Perform a natural release method.
7. Shred the pork and combine it with the juices, discard the bay leaves.
8. Add a bit more cumin and adobo if needed. Stir well and serve.

Pork Ribs

Prep Time: 10 min. Cook Time: 1 hr.
Yields: 6 Servings – 3 ribs.

Nutrition: 387 Cal., 27 g Prot., 29 g Fat, 2 g Net Carbs.
17 Smart Points.

Ingredients

- ✓ 1 (5 lb.) country style pork ribs

For the Rub
- ✓ 1 tbsp. erythritol/another sweetener
- ✓ 1 t. of each:
  - o Paprika
  - o Onion powder
  - o Garlic powder
- ✓ ½ t. of each:
  - o Black pepper
  - o Ground coriander
  - o Allspice

Ingredients for the Sauce

- ✓ 2 tbsp. of each:
  - o Erythritol/your favorite sweetener
  - o Red wine vinegar
- ✓ ½ c. reduced-sugar/homemade
- ✓ ¼ c. liquid smoke
- ✓ ½ c. water
- ✓ ½ t. onion powder
- ✓ ½ tbsp. ground of each:
  - o Allspice
  - o Mustard

¼ t. xanthan gum - optional

How to Make

1. Rub down the ribs with the combined seasonings and stack them in your Instant Pot.
2. Mix the sauce fixings and pour over the ribs.
3. Secure the lid and set for 35 minutes (manually) under high pressure.
4. Perform a natural release method and place the ribs in a container to keep warm.
5. Whisk in the xanthan gum (if needed) and cook the juices for ten minutes using the sauté function.
6. Serve and enjoy!

Pork Vegetables & Noodles

Prep Time: 5 min. Cooking Time: 15 min.
Yields: 6 Servings.

Nutrition: 241 Cal., 15 g Prot., 18 g Fat, 3 g Net Carbs.
11 Smart Points.

Ingredients
- ✓ 1 tbsp. oil
- ✓ 1 lb. ground pork
- ✓ 1 c. chopped bell peppers
- ✓ 2 garlic cloves
- ✓ ½ c. chopped onion
- ✓ 4 c. chopped baby spinach
- ✓ 2 pkg. shirataki noodles
- ✓ ½ c. grated parmesan cheese

How to Make
1. Prepare your Instant Pot using the sauté function and add the oil when hot.
2. Toss in the pork and sauté until slightly pink.
3. Add the garlic, onions, peppers and spinach.
4. Scrape the browning bits off the bottom and secure the lid.
5. Use the high-pressure setting to cook for three minutes.
6. Perform a quick release method.
7. Empty the sauce over the noodles and garnish with the cheese.

Leg of Lamb

Prep Time: 5 min. Cook Time: 35 min.
Yields: 8 Servings.

Nutrition: 432 Cal., 44.7 g Prot., 25.82 g Fat, 0.64 g Net Carbs. **16 Smart Points.**

Ingredients
- ✓ 1 boneless (3-4 lb.) leg of lamb
- ✓ 2 c. water
- ✓ 2 tbsp. avocado oil – divided
- ✓ 4 crushed garlic cloves
- ✓ Pepper & Salt to taste
- ✓ 2 tbsp. freshly chopped rosemary

How to Make
1. Dry the lamb using paper towels. Sprinkle with pepper and salt.
2. Use the sauté button to start the Instant Pot and add the oil.
3. When hot, place the lamb in the pot and brown.
4. Transfer the lamb to a platter and cover with the rosemary and crushed garlic.
5. Add the rack to the pot and arrange the lamb on it.
6. Pour in the water and select the meat/stew setting. Cook for 30-35 minutes (30 min. for med. rare).
7. Perform a natural release method.
8. Preheat the oven broiler and place the lamb on a pan about six inches from the heat. Two minutes should do the trick.
9. Let it rest for about ten minutes before slicing.
10. Serve and enjoy.

Mashed Potatoes

Prep Time: 10 min. Cook Time: 20 min.
Yields:6 Servings.

Nutrition: 98 Cal., 0 g Prot., 9.50 g Fat, 1 g Net Carbs.
6 Smart Points.

Ingredients

- ✓ 1 ½ c. water
- ✓ 5-6 baking potatoes
- ✓ ½ t. salt
- ✓ 5 garlic cloves
- ✓ 1 tbsp. vegan butter/extra-virgin olive oil
- ✓ Dash black pepper
- ✓ Pinch of nutmeg
- ✓ Dash of thyme/parsley
- ✓ 1 c. full-fat coconut milk
- ✓ For the Garnish: Fresh chives

How to Make

1. Add the garlic cloves, ¼ t. of salt, water, and the cubed potatoes into the Instant Pot. Set for four minutes on high pressure.
2. Perform a natural release method.
3. Drain well, mashing slightly to help cool.
4. Mince the garlic and add it to the rest of the ingredients, salt, and ½ cup of the coconut milk (more if needed). Whip lightly for texture and let it rest.
5. Taste and adjust the salt as needed.
6. Top it off with some chives and serve.

Vegetarian Butter Chicken with Soy Curls

Prep Time: 5 min. Cook Time:15 min.
Yields:6 Servings.

Nutrition: 254 Cal., 5 g Prot., 24 g Fat, 4 g Net Carbs.
14 Smart Points.

Ingredients

- ✓ 1 c. water
- ✓ 1 ½ cups dry soy curls
- ✓ 1 can (14.5 oz.) diced tomatoes
- ✓ 5-6 garlic cloves
- ✓ ½ t. cayenne pepper
- ✓ 1 t. of each:
    - o Ground cumin
    - o Garam masala
    - o Paprika
    - o Salt
    - o Turmeric
    - o Cayenne pepper
- ✓ 1-2 t. minced ginger

How to Make

1. Add the fixings (water, spices, soy curls, and tomatoes) and cook for 6 minutes under high pressure.
2. Perform a natural release method for ten minutes and follow with a quick release.
3. Switch your pot to the sauté function and add the butter.
4. Garnish as you like and enjoy.

Lazy Devils

This recipe needs 4 minutes of preparation, 16 minutes of cooking time and will make 8 servings.

Nutrition: 32 Cal., 2.2g Fat, 2.8g Protein, 0.3g Net Carbs.
1 Smart Points.

Ingredients

- ✓ 8 eggs -large
- ✓ 8 radishes - sliced
- ✓ 1/2 c. guacamole
- ✓ Salt and ground pepper to taste
- ✓ 1 c. water

How to Make

1. Add the water and eggs to your Instant Pot. Lock the lid, close the valve, and press Manual / High for 6 minutes on the timer.
2. Manually vent the pressure and carefully remove the eggs. Let them cool before peeling.
3. Slice the eggs in half and separate the yolks.
4. Add the yolks, guacamole, salt and pepper. Smash the yolks with a fork and mix well.
5. Spoon the mixture into the eggs, top with radish and serve. Or chill for a later snack.

Japanese Turkey Meatballs

This recipe needs 15 minutes of preparation, 15 minutes of cooking time and will make 4 servings.

Nutrition: 185 Cal., 0.4g Fat, 23g Protein, 2g Net Carbs.
3 Smart Points.

Ingredients

- ✓ 1 pound ground turkey meat
- ✓ 1/4 c. water
- ✓ 2T fresh cilantro - chopped
- ✓ 1/2 t. each:
  - o White Pepper
  - o Sea Salt
- ✓ 2/3 t. onion powder
- ✓ 1 T soy sauce
- ✓ 2 t. sesame oil
- ✓ 1/2 red chili - diced fine

How to Make

1. In a large bowl, mix all the ingredients except for the water.
2. Wet your hands and roll the mixture into small meatballs.
3. Add the water and steamer into your Instant Pot.
4. Set the meatballs in the steamer, lock the lid, close the valve and press Manual / High for 7 minutes on the timer.
5. Manually vent the pressure, remove the steamer and set the meatballs aside.
6. Empty any remaining water and turn your Instant Pot to Sauté mode. Add the meatballs and allow them to brown on each side for about a minute.
7. Remove and serve or refrigerate for snacks later.

Cauliflower & Cheese

Prep Time: 5 min. Cook Time: 15 min.
Yields: 4 Servings.

Nutrition: 134 Cal., 2g Prot., 10g Fat, 5g Net Carbs.
7 Smart Points.

Ingredients
- ✓ 2 tbsp. cream cheese
- ✓ 2 c. riced cauliflower
- ✓ Salt & Pepper – to taste
- ✓ ½ c. of each:
  - o Half & Half
  - o Shredded sharp cheddar cheese
- ✓ 1 ½ c. water

How to Make
1. Combine all the ingredients in a heat-proof bowl.
2. Cover with foil.
3. Pour the water into the Instant Pot. Add the bowl on a trivet in the pot.
4. Set the timer for five minutes under high pressure.
5. Perform a natural release method for ten minutes, then perform a quick release method to release the remaining steam.
6. Warm up the oven broiler and add the cauliflower on the rack to brown the cheese. Serve when bubbly.

Cauliflower Soufflé

Prep Time: 10 min. Cook Time: 22 min.
Yields: 6 Servings.

Nutrition: 342 Cal., 17 g Prot., 28 g Fat, 5 g Net Carbs.
16 Smart Points.

Ingredients
- ✓ 2 eggs
- ✓ 1 head cauliflower
- ✓ ½ c. of each:
  - o Asiago cheese
  - o Sour cream/Yogurt
- ✓ 2 tbsp. cream
- ✓ 2 oz. cream cheese
- ✓ 1 c. mild/sharp cheddar cheese
- ✓ 2 t. softened butter/ghee
- ✓ ¼ c. chives
- ✓ Optional: 6 slices crumbled cooked bacon

How to Make
1. Combine the two kinds of cheese, sour cream, cream cheese, cream and eggs in a food processor. Pulse until smooth and frothy.
2. Chop the cauliflower and add it to the mixture (pulse 2 seconds at a time).
3. Blend in the butter and chives. Empty them into a 1 ¼ quart casserole dish.
4. Pour the water into the Instant Pot. Secure the top and cook for 12 minutes using the high-pressure setting.
5. Perform a natural release method for ten minutes, and then perform a quick release method to release the remaining steam.
6. Garnish and serve with bacon if you choose.

Spaghetti Squash

Prep Time: 2 min. Cook Time: 13 min.
Yields: 2 Servings.

Nutrition: 90Cal., 10g Prot., 5g Fat, 3g Net Carbs.
3 Smart Points.

Ingredients
- ✓ 1 c. cold water
- ✓ 1 whole spaghetti squash – 3 lb. approx.

How to Make
1. Slice the squash in half – lengthwise. Dispose of the seeds.
2. Add the steamer rack and one cup of water into the Instant Pot.
3. Arrange the squash on the rack and secure the lid.
4. Use high pressure for six minutes and quick release for eight minutes for softer squash.
5. Open the top and transfer the squash to a container.
6. Gently remove the flesh and remove the 'spaghetti-like' strands. Serve.

Black Bean Dip

This recipe needs 15 minutes to prepare, 30 minutes to cook and will prepare enough black bean dip for 24 servings.

Protein: 8.3g. Net Carbs: 2.5g. Fat: 18.7g. Calories: 201.
10 Smart Points.

Ingredients
- ✓ Black Beads (1.5 C or 375mL, dried)
- ✓ Onion (1 C or 250mL, diced)
- ✓ Paprika (1 TSP)
- ✓ Garlic (4 cloves, minced)
- ✓ Jalapeno (.33 C or 90mL, diced)
- ✓ Sea Salt (.75 TSP)
- ✓ Crushed Tomatoes (15oz can)
- ✓ Vegetable Broth (1.75 C or 440mL)
- ✓ Cumin (2 TSP)
- ✓ Lime Juice (from 1 lime)
- ✓ Chili Powder (.5 TSP)
- ✓ Ground Coriander (.5 TSP)

How to Make
1. Thoroughly rinse your black beans before placing them in your instant pot.
2. Add all the remaining ingredients and blend thoroughly.
3. Manually set your instant pot to a high pressure setting.
4. Cook the bean dip for 30 minutes.
5. Perform a natural release method until your instant pot has released its pressure over 10 minutes.
6. When your instant pot has been releasing for 10 minutes, perform a quick release method as outlined in your instant pot's user manual.
7. Transfer the contents into your blender and blend until creamy and smooth.
8. Serve & Enjoy!

Southwestern Spicy Spinach Dip

This recipe needs 5 minutes to prepare, 20 minutes to cook, and will make enough to serve 10 servings.

Protein: 13.1g. Net Carbs: 5.7g. Fat: 22.3g. Calories: 269. **13 Smart Points.**

Ingredients

- ✓ Spinach (1lb)
- ✓ Sour Cream (.25 C or 75mL)
- ✓ Half and Half (.25 C or 75mL)
- ✓ Tomatoes (3 medium, finely chopped)
- ✓ Garlic (5 cloves, minced)
- ✓ Ground Cumin (1 TSP)
- ✓ Cheddar Cheese (1 C or 250mL, grated)
- ✓ Mozzarella Cheese (1 C or 250mL, grated)
- ✓ Cream Cheese (4oz, cubed)
- ✓ Olive Oil (1 T)
- ✓ Onion Powder (1 TSP)
- ✓ Jalapenos (2, seeded and minced)
- ✓ Chili Powder (1 TSP)
- ✓ Hot Sauce (1 T)
- ✓ Black Olives (.5 C or 125mL)

How to Make

1. Begin by sautéing the spinach, garlic and tomatoes in your instant pot.
2. Cook until the spinach is wilted. Turn off your instant pot.
3. Add all the dairy products, olives, jalapenos, hot sauce and spices into your instant pot and manually set it to high pressure. Cook for 4 minutes.
4. Perform a quick release method to release the pressure as outlined in your manufacturer's guide.
5. Season with salt and pepper if desired.
6. Serve & enjoy!

Cheeseburger Dip

This recipe needs 5 minutes to prepare, 20 minutes to cook, and will prepare enough cheeseburger dip for 10 servings.

Protein: 8.3g. Net Carbs: 2.5g. Fats: 18.7g. Calories: 201. **10 Smart Points.**

Ingredients

- ✓ Ground Beef (.5lb)
- ✓ Diced Tomatoes (10oz can)
- ✓ Cheddar Cheese (1 C or 250mL, grated)
- ✓ Cream Cheese (8oz, cubed)
- ✓ Water (4 T)
- ✓ Bacon (4-5 slices, cut into half-inch pieces)

How to Make

1. Sauté the bacon in your instant pot until it is cooked but not crispy.
2. Place it on a paper-towel lined plate to rest for now.
3. Cook the ground beef until it is completely browned, then add water, bacon and cream cheese into the pot. Do not stir the ingredients together, rather let them sit as-is.
4. Seal the lid and manually set the instant pot to high pressure.
5. Cook the dip for 4 minutes.
6. Perform a quick release on your instant pot as per your manufacturer's guidelines.
7. Add the remaining cheeses and stir consistently until the cream cheese chunks have dissolved and the entire dip is creamy.
8. Serve and enjoy.

Sweet Fire Hot Wings

This recipe needs 5 minutes of preparation, 25 minutes of cooking time and will make 6 servings.

Nutrition: 595 Cal., 22.4g Fat, 87.5g Protein, 5.3g Net Carbs. **16 Smart Points.**

Ingredients

- ✓ 4 pounds chicken wings - fat trimmed
- ✓ 1/2 c. each coconut sugar, Paleo wing sauce, and water
- ✓ Kosher salt and fresh ground pepper to taste
- ✓ 1/2 c. water

How to Make

1. Season wings with salt/pepper. Toss until well coated. Insert a trivet into your Instant Pot. Pour in water.
2. Place the wings on a trivet.
3. Place a lid on your pot and close the vent. Set the Manual button on high and set the timer for 5 minutes.
4. Preheat your instant pot using the Broil function.
5. Cover a baking sheet with foil and set a cooling rack sprayed with nonstick spray on top.
6. Combine sugar and wing sauce into a microwavable safe bowl. Microwave on High for one minute. Stir and if the sugar is not completely melted, repeat for an additional 15 seconds.
7. When the timer is complete on your Instant Pot, let the pressure vent naturally for 10 minutes and then use the quick-release method. Remove the lid.
8. Place the wings in a large bowl and use half the wing sauce mixture to completely cover the wings.
9. Place the wings on a wire rack and set in the oven. Leave the door vented.
10. After 5 minutes, flip the wings and rotate the sheet halfway and place back it back into the oven for 5 minutes.
11. Remove the wings and add them back into the bowl. Pour the remaining sauce over the chicken and toss well.
12. Serve immediately.

Spicy BBQ Wings

This recipe needs 5 minutes of preparation, 25 minutes of cooking time and will make 6 servings.

Nutrition: 710 Cal., 25.2g Fat, 87.6g Protein, 24.4g Net Carbs. **20 Smart Points.**

Ingredients

- ✓ 4 pounds chicken wings - fat trimmed
- ✓ 3/4 c. Paleo BBQ sauce
- ✓ 2 jalapeño peppers - diced finely
- ✓ 1/2 c. water
- ✓ Kosher salt and fresh ground pepper to taste

How to Make

1. Season the wings with salt and pepper. Toss them around until well coated.
2. Insert a trivet into your Instant Pot. Pour in water and place the wings on a trivet.
3. Place a lid on your pot and close the vent.
4. Select the Manual button and High. Set timer for 5 minutes.
5. Preheat your pot using the Broil mode.
6. Cover a baking sheet with foil and set a cooling rack sprayed with nonstick spray on top.
7. Let the pressure vent naturally for 10 minutes and then perform a quick-release method. Remove the lid.
8. Place the wings in a large bowl and use half of the BBQ sauce to completely cover them and then sprinkle with the diced peppers—for spicier wings add the peppers, seeds and juices to the BBQ sauce and stir well before coating wings.
9. Place the wings on a wire rack and set in the oven.
10. After 5 minutes, flip the wings, rotate the sheet halfway and place it back into the oven for 5 minutes.
11. Remove the wings and add them back into the bowl. Pour the remaining BBQ sauce over chicken and toss well.
12. Serve immediately.

Coconut Almond Cake

Prep Time: 10 min. Cook Time: 40 min.
Yields: 8 Servings.

Nutrition: 236 Cal., 5 g Prot., 23 g Fat, 3 g Net Carbs.
15 Smart Points.

Dry Ingredients
- ✓ 1 c. almond flour
- ✓ ½ c. unsweetened shredded coconut
- ✓ 1/3 c. Truvia
- ✓ 1 t. of each:
    - ○ Apple pie spice
    - ○ Baking powder

Wet Ingredients
- ✓ ¼ c. melted butter
- ✓ 2 lightly whisked eggs
- ✓ ½ c. heavy whipping cream

Also Needed
- ✓ 1 (6-inch) round cake pan.
- ✓ 2 c. water

How to Make
1. Combine all the dry ingredients together inside a bowl. Add each of the 'wet' ingredients – one at a time.
2. Empty the batter into the pan and cover it with foil.
3. Empty the water into the Instant Pot and place the steamer rack.
4. Set the timer for 40 minutes using the high-pressure setting.
5. Perform a natural release method for 10 minutes. Then, perform a quick release method.
6. Remove the pan and let it cool 15 to 20 minutes.
7. Flip it over onto a platter and garnish as desired (count the carbs).

Peanut Butter Chocolate Cheesecake

Prep Time: 5 min. Cooking Time: 18 min.
Yields: 8 Servings.

Nutrition: 191 Cal., 6 g Prot., 16 g Fat, 5 g Net Carbs.
14 Smart Points.

Ingredients
- ✓ 2 eggs
- ✓ 16 oz. cheese
- ✓ 2 tbsp. powdered peanut butter
- ✓ 1 t. vanilla extract
- ✓ 1 tbsp. cocoa
- ✓ ½ c. sugar substitute of choice

How to Make
1. Let all the ingredients come to room temperature.
2. Toss the eggs and cream cheese into the blender. Mix until smooth.
3. Add the remainder of the components and blend them well.
4. Add the mixture into 4 (4 ounce) mason jars and cover with some aluminum foil or jar lid.
5. Pour one cup of water into your Instant Pot. You will need to prepare them in two batches.
6. Cook on high for 15 to 18 minutes.
7. Perform a natural release method and chill overnight or at least several hours.
8. Serve and enjoy!

Ricotta Lemon Cheesecake

Prep Time: 10 min. Cook Time: 40 min.
Yields: 6 Servings.

Nutrition: 181 Cal., 5g Prot., 16g Fat, 2g Net Carbs.
11 Smart Points.

Ingredients
- ✓ 8 oz. cream cheese
- ✓ ¼ c. Truvia
- ✓ 1 lemon – Zest and juice
- ✓ 1/3 c. Ricotta cheese
- ✓ ½ t. lemon extract
- ✓ 2 eggs

Ingredients for the Topping
- ✓ 1 t. Truvia
- ✓ 2 tbsp. sour cream

Also Needed:
- ✓ A 6-inch springform pan

How to Make
1. Combine all the ingredients in a stand mixer (except for the eggs).
2. Taste test and add the eggs. Use a low speed, since over-beating the eggs will cause the crust to crack.
3. Add the batter to the pan. Cover with foil/silicone lid.
4. Add the trivet and two cups of water and arrange the pan in the Instant Pot.
5. Cook for 30 minutes on high-pressure.
6. Perform a natural release method.
7. Blend in the Truvia and sour cream.
8. Decorate the warm cake and place it into the fridge to chill for six to eight hours.

Thai Coconut Pandan Custard

Prep Time: 10 mins Cook Time: 30 mins Yields: 4 Servings.

Nutrition: 174 Cal., 6 g Prot., 14 g Fat, 6 g Net Carbs.
12 Smart Points.

Ingredients
- ✓ 3 eggs
- ✓ 1 c. unsweetened coconut milk
- ✓ 1/3 c. Truvia baking blend/favorite sweetener
- ✓ 3-4 drops vanilla extract/Pandan Extract
- ✓ 2 c. water

How to Make
1. Combine the sweetener, eggs and Pandan Extract together into a heat-proof (6-inch) bowl. Place foil over the top.
2. Pour the water into the Instant Pot and add the trivet. Put the bowl in the center of the pot. Set the timer for 30 minutes using high pressure.
3. Perform a natural release method.
4. Check when the custard is set with a knife—ensuring it comes out clean.
5. Cool the custard in the fridge until chilled and completely set.

Cheese Popcorn

Prep Time: 3 min. - Cooking Time: 5 min.
Yields: 6 Servings.

Nutrition: 154.4 Calories, 10.5 g Protein, 10.7 g Fat, 4.1 g Net Carbs. **8 Smart Points.**

Ingredients
- ✓ 1 tbsp. garlic puree
- ✓ ½ c. corn
- ✓ 1 ¼ c. cheddar cheese
- ✓ 2 t. coconut oil
- ✓ Salt to taste

How to Make
1. Select the sauté function and add the coconut oil in your instant pot.
2. When melted, add in the salt, garlic and corn. Stir until coated.
3. Place the cover on the Instant Pot (no need to seal).
4. After the corn pops two to three minutes; turn off the power.
5. When popping is complete, add the grated cheese and wait for it to melt.
6. Enjoy every morsel!

Crust-less Cheesecake

Prep time: 15 minutes - Cooking time: 20 minutes
Yields: 4-6 servings.

Nutrition: 421 Cal., 28 g Fat, 12 g Prot., 2 g Net Carbs. **20 Smart Points.**

Ingredients
- ✓ Big handful of fresh strawberries
- ✓ 2 room temp eggs
- ✓ 1 tsp. vanilla extract
- ✓ 2/3 C. sugar substitute of choice
- ✓ 2 8-ounce blocks of full-fat cream cheese

How to make
1. Grease a springform pan.
2. Blend the cream cheese with a hand mixer till it is smooth.
3. Mix the vanilla and sugar substitute with cream cheese until it is well incorporated.
4. Add the eggs, mixing them in one at a time. Be careful not to over mix them.
5. Pour the batter into the pan. Cover the sides and bottom with foil so that water doesn't leak into it.
6. Put the rack into the bottom of the instant pot.
7. Add just enough water to cover the bottom.
8. Place the springform pan into the instant pot.
9. Cook on MANUAL and HIGH for 20 minutes.

Keto Coconut Almond Cake

Prep time: 10 minutes - Cooking time: 40 minutes
Yields: 6-8 servings.

Nutrition: 489 Cal., 26 g Fat, 14 g Prot., 4 g Net Carbs.
22 Smart Points.

Ingredients
- ✓ 1 tsp. apple pie spice
- ✓ 1 tsp. baking powder
- ✓ 1/3 C. Truvia
- ✓ ½ C. unsweetened shredded coconut
- ✓ 1 C. almond flour
- ✓ ½ C. heavy whipping cream
- ✓ ¼ C. melted butter
- ✓ 2 lightly whisked eggs

How to make
1. Combine all the dry recipe components.
2. Mix together all the wet recipe ingredients, and then stir in with dry mixture. Pour into round cake pan.
3. Pour 2 cups of water into bottom of your instant pot and place a steamer rack inside. Place a cake pan on the top.
4. Press HIGH to cook for 40 minutes.
5. perform a natural release for 10 minutes, then release any pressure remaining manually.
6. Take out the pan and allow it to cool for at least 20 minutes.
7. Sprinkle with powdered sweetener, almonds and more shredded coconut if desired.

Dark Chocolate Walnut Cake

Prep time: 10 minutes - Cooking time: 20 minutes
Yields: 8 servings.

Nutrition: 311 Cal., 17 g Fat, 7 g Prot., 2 g Net Carbs.
15 Smart Points.

Ingredients
- ✓ ¼ C. coconut oil
- ✓ 1/3 C. heavy whipping cream
- ✓ 3 eggs
- ✓ 1 tsp. baking powder
- ✓ ¼ C. chopped walnuts
- ✓ ¼ C. unsweetened cocoa powder
- ✓ 2/3 C. Swerve
- ✓ 1 C. almond flour

How to make
1. Grease a cake pan.
2. With a hand mixer, mix all the recipe components until fluffy.
3. Pour the cake batter into the pan.
4. Pour 2 cups of water into the bottom of your instant pot and place the steamer rack over the water.
5. Place a cake pan on the rack.
6. Set on HIGH and cook for 20 minutes.
7. Perform a natural pressure release method for 10 minutes.
8. Devour!

Almond Carrot Cake

Prep time: 10 minutes - Cooking time: 40 minutes
Yields: 6-8 servings.

Nutrition: 367 Cal., 19 g Fat, 8 g Prot., 1 g Net Carbs.
16 Smart Points.

Ingredients

- ✓ ½ C. walnuts
- ✓ 1 C. shredded carrots
- ✓ ½ C. heavy whipping cream
- ✓ ¼ C. coconut oil
- ✓ 1 ½ tsp. apple pie spice
- ✓ 1 tsp. baking powder
- ✓ 2/3 C. Swerve
- ✓ 1 C. almond flour
- ✓ 3 eggs

How to make

1. Grease a cake pan.
2. Combine all the ingredients with a hand mixer until it looks fluffy.
3. Pour them into a pan and cover it with foil.
4. Pour 2 cups of water into the instant pot and put a trivet over the water.
5. Place a cake pan onto the trivet.
6. Set to HIGH and cook 40 minutes.
7. Allow a natural pressure release for 10 minutes.
8. Allow it to cool before frosting it with your choice of frosting.
9. Enjoy!

Chocolate Pudding Cake

Prep time: 20 minutes - Cooking time: 5 minutes
Yields: 2 servings.

Nutrition: 287 Cal., 15 g Fat, 4 g Prot., 1 g Net Carbs.
14 Smart Points.

Ingredients

- ✓ 3 tbsp. cocoa powder
- ✓ ¼ C. arrowroot
- ✓ Pinch of salt
- ✓ 1 tsp. vanilla extract
- ✓ 2 eggs
- ✓ ½ C. applesauce
- ✓ 2/3 C. semi-sweet chocolate morsels

How to make

1. Put a trivet into your instant pot and pour in 2 cups water.
2. Pour the morsels into a ramekin and place it on the trivet.
3. Set your instant pot to SAUTE and melt the chocolate over the water.
4. Remove the ramekin when the chocolate melts.
5. Mix the vanilla, eggs and applesauce together. Then add cocoa powder, salt and combine well.
6. Then stir in the melted chocolate.
7. Grease a cake pan with coconut oil.
8. Dust the bottom and sides of the pan with cocoa powder.
9. Pour the cake batter into a pan and set the pan on top of a trivet inside your instant pot.
10. Cook on HIGH for 4 minutes.
11. Perform a quick release method
12. Take out the cake and allow it to cool for 10 minutes before putting on a serving platter.
13. Dust with powdered sugar if you choose. Devour!

Applesauce

This recipe needs 10 minutes of preparation, 10 minutes of cooking time and will make 10 servings.

Nutrition: 145 Cal., 0.5g Fat, 0.7g Protein, 38.4g Net Carbs. **6 Smart Points.**

Ingredients

- ✓ 12 apples - peeled, cored, and diced
- ✓ 1/2 c. apple cider

How to Make

1. Add the ingredients to your Instant Pot.
2. Place a piece of parchment paper over the apples.
3. Lock the lid, close the valve and select Manual / High for 10 minutes on the timer.
4. Let the pressure vent naturally, discard the paper and remove the apples.
5. In a food processor or blender, blend until smooth. Refrigerate for a great snack throughout the week.

Mini Crust Less Pumpkin Pie

This recipe needs 5 minutes of preparation, 15 minutes of cooking time and will make 8 servings.

Nutrition: 143.9 Cal., 2.3g Fat, 3.3g Protein, 29.1g Net Carbs. **6 Smart Points.**

Ingredients

- ✓ 2 pounds butternut squash - peeled and diced
- ✓ 1 c. coconut milk
- ✓ 3/4 c. pure maple syrup
- ✓ 2 large eggs
- ✓ 1/4 t. powdered cloves
- ✓ 1/2 t. powdered ginger
- ✓ 1 t. powdered cinnamon
- ✓ 1 T organic cornstarch
- ✓ 2 pinches Sea Salt
- ✓ 1 c. water

How to Make

1. Add 1 c. water and steamer basket to your Instant Pot.
2. Add squash cubes to steamer basket, lock lid, close valve, hit Manual / High, and add 4 minutes on the timer and manually vent pressure when done.
3. In a medium mixing bowl, add milk, maple syrup, eggs, cinnamon, ginger, salt, and cornstarch. Beat well.
4. Tumble squash in a fine-mesh strainer and when cooled, press on the pulp to drain liquid.
5. Pour 2 c. of juice into the egg mixture and mix well - discard remainder or freeze for stock.
6. If needed, add additional water to Instant Pot and insert trivet.
7. Pour mixture into heat-proof ramekins and place on a trivet, stacking ramekins as needed.
8. Lock lid, close valve, hit Manual / High, and add 10 minutes on the timer and let pressure vent naturally when done.
9. Let stand 5 minutes before serving. Let cool completely, cover tightly and refrigerate for up to two days for another great Paleo snack for later.

Blueberry Jam

This recipe needs 20 minutes of preparation, 30 minutes of cooking time and will make between 3 and 5 half-pint jars.

Nutrition: 95 Cal., 0.2g Fat, 0.4g Protein, 25.3g Net Carbs.
5 Smart Points.

Ingredients
- ✓ 2 pounds fresh blueberries
- ✓ 1-pound local honey

How to Make
1. Add the ingredients into your Instant Pot and turn to Low until the honey melts.
2. Press the Sauté mode on your pot and let the mixture come to a boil, stirring often.
3. Lock the lid, close the valve and press the Manual / High button for 2 minutes on the timer.
4. Perform a natural release method.
5. Turn your Instant Pot back to Sauté mode and bring to a boil again, stirring often and completely deglazing the bottom of the pan until some of the liquid evaporates and the jam is a nice consistency.
6. Spoon the jam into jars and store it in the refrigerator.

Tapioca Pudding

This recipe needs 5 minutes of preparation, 15 minutes of cooking time and will make 8 servings.

Nutrition: 138 Cal., 3.1g Fat, 0.3g Protein, 27.2g Net Carbs.
7 Smart Points.

Ingredients
- ✓ 1 can full-fat coconut milk
- ✓ 1/3 c. small tapioca pearls
- ✓ 1/4 c. maple syrup
- ✓ 1 t. vanilla extract
- ✓ 1 pinch sea salt
- ✓ 1 c. water
- ✓ 1/4 t. ground nutmeg

How to Make
1. Add water and a steamer basket inside your Instant Pot.
2. Combine all the ingredients in a heat-proof bowl and mix well.
3. Place a bowl in the steamer, lock the lid, close the valve and press Manual / High for 20 minutes on the timer.
4. Perform a quick-release method.
5. Stir the mixture and move the bowl to the fridge to chill for 1 hour or until a desired thickness.
6. Serve or spoon into small jars for a great snack later.

Banana Bread

This recipe needs 5 minutes of preparation, 30 minutes of cooking time and will make 6 servings.

Nutrition: 151 Cal., 12.3g Fat, 1.5g Protein, 9.9g Net Carbs.
10 Smart Points.

Ingredients

- ✓ 1/3 c. cashew or almond milk
- ✓ 2 very ripe bananas - mashed
- ✓ 3/4 c. coconut sugar
- ✓ 1 egg - room temperature
- ✓ 1 1/2 tsp cream of tartar
- ✓ 1 t. vanilla
- ✓ 1 1/2 c. Cassava flour
- ✓ 1 tsp baking powder
- ✓ 1/2 tsp baking soda
- ✓ pinch of salt
- ✓ 1/3 c. softened ghee
- ✓ 2 c. water

How to Make

1. In a small bowl, mix the milk and cream of tartar and set it aside.
2. In another bowl, add the butter, sugar, egg and vanilla. Mix well.
3. Add the bananas and continue to mix.
4. In another separate bowl, mix the flour, baking powder, baking soda and salt. Gradually add dry ingredients while mixing.
5. Add the milk mixture, stir and pour into a small greased cake pan and cover with foil.
6. Add water and the trivet to your Instant Pot and place the cake pan on the trivet.
7. Lock the lid, close the valve, and press Manual / High for 30 minutes on the timer.
8. Perform a natural release method.
9. Carefully remove the pan, uncover, and allow the cake to cool on a wire rack.
10. Serve and enjoy.

Apple Crisp

This recipe needs 5 minutes of preparation, 8 minutes of cooking time and will make 4 servings.

Nutrition: 219 Cal., 1.5g Fat, 2.8g Protein, 53.2Net Carbs.
8 Smart Points.

Ingredients

- ✓ 5 medium apples - peeled and Chopped
- ✓ 3/4 c. Steel Cut Oats
- ✓ 1 T maple syrup
- ✓ 1/4 c. coconut sugar
- ✓ 2 t. cinnamon
- ✓ 1/2 t. nutmeg
- ✓ 4T Paleo butter - melted
- ✓ 1/4c. Paleo flour
- ✓ 1/2 t. salt
- ✓ 1/2 c. water

How to Make

1. Pour water into your Instant Pot. Add the apples. Coat with cinnamon and nutmeg. Top with maple syrup.
2. In small bowl, mix the butter, salt, brown sugar, oats and flour.
3. Spoon the mixture on top of the apples.
4. Place the lid on the pot and close the vent.
5. Select the Manual / High setting and set the timer for 8 minutes.
6. When timer completes, allow the pressure to vent naturally.
7. The mixture will thicken as it stands.
8. Serve warm.

Pumpkin Chocolate Chip Bundt Cake

This recipe needs 12 minutes of preparation, 45 minutes of cooking time and will make 12 servings.

Nutrition: 194 Cal., 44.5g Fat, 43.2g Protein, 170.2g Net Carbs. **16 Smart Points.**

Ingredients

- ✓ 1 medium banana- mashed
- ✓ 1/2 can pumpkin - 7.5 ounces
- ✓ 1 medium egg
- ✓ 1/2 c. Greek yogurt
- ✓ 1 1/2 c. Paleo Flour
- ✓ 1/2 t. each salt and baking powder
- ✓ 1 t. baking soda
- ✓ 3/4 t. pumpkin pie spice
- ✓ 3/4 c.coconut sugar
- ✓ ½ t. pure vanilla extract
- ✓ 2/3 c. Paleo chocolate chips
- ✓ 2T coconut oil
- ✓ 1 1/2 c. water

How to Make

1. In a medium bowl, combine the pumpkin pie spice, baking powder, flour, salt and baking soda. Set aside.
2. In a medium mixing bowl, add the pumpkin, banana, sugar, egg, vanilla, yogurt and oil. Use an electric mixer to combine well.
3. Turn the mixer to low and slowly add the dry ingredient mixture. Mix well.
4. Fold in the chocolate chips.
5. Spray the Bundt pan with nonstick spray and pour in the batter.
6. Cover the pan with a layer of paper towels and then cover with foil.
7. Add water to the Instant Pot and insert the trivet.
8. Place the Bundt pan in the Instant Pot.
9. Place the lid on the pot and close the vent.
10. Select the Manual / High setting and set the timer for 35 minutes.
11. When the timer completes, allow the pressure to vent naturally for 10 minutes.
12. Perform the quick release method.
13. Remove the lid and let the pan cool for a few minutes before removing.

Baked Apples

This recipe needs 5 minutes of preparation, 20 minutes of cooking time and will make 6 servings.

Nutrition: 189 Cal., 0.3g Fat, 0.6g Protein, 41.9g Net Carbs. **8 Smart Points.**

Ingredients

- ✓ 6 fresh apples - cored
- ✓ 1/2 c. coconut sugar
- ✓ 1/4 c. raisins
- ✓ 1 c. red wine
- ✓ 1 t. cinnamon powder

How to Make

1. Add the apples, wine, raisins, sugar and cinnamon to your Instant Pot.
2. Place the lid on the pot and close the vent.
3. Select the Manual / High setting and set the timer for 10 minutes.
4. When the timer completes, perform the quick-release method to vent pressure.
5. Serve and enjoy!

Lemon Cheesecake

This recipe needs 10 minutes to prepare, 40 minutes to cook, and will make enough lemon cheese cake for 6 servings.

Protein: 5g, Net Carbs: 2g, Fat: 16g Calories: 181.
11 Smart Points.

What to Use:

- ✓ Sweetener (.25 C or 75mL)
- ✓ Cream Cheese (8oz)
- ✓ Lemon Zest
- ✓ Ricotta Cheese (.33 C or 90mL)
- ✓ Lemon Extract (.5 TSP)
- ✓ Eggs (2 large)
- ✓ Sour Cream (2 T)

What to Do:

1. Combine all the ingredients except for the sour cream and eggs into a bowl.
2. Blend until they are completely smooth and free of clumps.
3. Add the eggs and blend – but not too much! Do not overbeat or the cheesecake will not cook properly.
4. Pour the ingredients into a small greased cake pan and cover them with foil so that any condensation does not ruin the cheesecake.
5. Pour two cups of water into the inner liner of your instant pot and fit it with a trivet. Place the cake pan on the trivet.
6. Manually set your instant pot to high pressure and cook for 30 minutes.
7. Perform a natural release method.
8. After, remove the cheesecake from the instant pot and cover with sour cream while it is still warm.
9. Place the cheesecake into the fridge and allow it to chill for 6-8 hours before serving.

Thai Coconut Custard

This recipe needs 5 minutes to prepare, 30 minutes to cook, and will prepare enough coconut custard for 4 servings.

Protein: 6g, Net Carbs: 6g, Fat: 14g, Calories: 174.
10 Smart Points.

What to Use:

- ✓ Eggs (3 large)
- ✓ Unsweetened Coconut Milk (1 C or 250mL)
- ✓ Swerve (.33 C or 90mL)

What to Do:

1. Begin by blending together all the ingredients.
2. Then, pour them into a heat-safe dish and cover the dish with foil.
3. In the inner liner of your instant pot, pour 2 cups of water.
4. Fit it with a trivet, then place the heat-proof dish inside the instant pot.
5. Manually set it to high pressure and cook for 30 minutes.
6. Then, allow the pressure to completely release naturally (do not use the quick release method!) This is how the custard will set.
7. Remove the dish from the instant pot and allow it to come to room temperature before transferring it into the fridge.
8. Allow it to cool completely until the custard is set.
9. Serve & enjoy!

Made in the USA
Middletown, DE
17 July 2018